Dear Future Exam Success Story:

Congratulations on your purchase of our study guide. Our goal in writing our study guide was to cover the content on the test, as well as provide insight into typical test taking mistakes and how to overcome them.

Standardized tests are a key component of being successful, which only increases the importance of doing well in the high-pressure high-stakes environment of test day. How well you do on this test will have a significant impact on your future, and we have the research and practical advice to help you execute on test day.

The product you're reading now is designed to exploit weaknesses in the test itself, and help you avoid the most common errors test takers frequently make.

How to use this study guide

We don't want to waste your time. Our study guide is fast-paced and fluff-free. We suggest going through it a number of times, as repetition is an important part of learning new information and concepts.

First, read through the study guide completely to get a feel for the content and organization. Read the general success strategies first, and then proceed to the content sections. Each tip has been carefully selected for its effectiveness.

Second, read through the study guide again, and take notes in the margins and highlight those sections where you may have a particular weakness.

Finally, bring the manual with you on test day and study it before the exam begins.

Your success is our success

We would be delighted to hear about your success. Send us an email and tell us your story. Thanks for your business and we wish you continued success.

Sincerely,
Mometrix Test Preparation Team

Need more help? Check out our flashcards at: http://MometrixFlashcards.com/NBCHPN

TABLE OF CONTENTS

Top 20 Test Taking Tips

1. Carefully follow all the test registration procedures
2. Know the test directions, duration, topics, question types, how many questions
3. Setup a flexible study schedule at least 3-4 weeks before test day
4. Study during the time of day you are most alert, relaxed, and stress free
5. Maximize your learning style; visual learner use visual study aids, auditory learner use auditory study aids
6. Focus on your weakest knowledge base
7. Find a study partner to review with and help clarify questions
8. Practice, practice, practice
9. Get a good night's sleep; don't try to cram the night before the test
10. Eat a well balanced meal
11. Know the exact physical location of the testing site; drive the route to the site prior to test day
12. Bring a set of ear plugs; the testing center could be noisy
13. Wear comfortable, loose fitting, layered clothing to the testing center; prepare for it to be either cold or hot during the test
14. Bring at least 2 current forms of ID to the testing center
15. Arrive to the test early; be prepared to wait and be patient
16. Eliminate the obviously wrong answer choices, then guess the first remaining choice
17. Pace yourself; don't rush, but keep working and move on if you get stuck
18. Maintain a positive attitude even if the test is going poorly
19. Keep your first answer unless you are positive it is wrong
20. Check your work, don't make a careless mistake

Certified Hospice and Palliative Nursing Assistant

Patient and Family Care

Activities of daily living

Activities of Daily Living (ADL) are the activities people perform routinely that allow independent living.

- *Hygiene:* Preparation for bathing (undressing and assembling all necessary gear); the ability to bath or shower; and getting in and out of the tub or shower stall.
- *Mobility:* The ability to transfer from one place to another, as from the bed to a chair, and moving from one place to another.
- *Nutrition:* Preparing food and drink; putting the food and drink into the mouth; chewing and swallowing solids and liquids.
- *Grooming:* The ability to dress and undress.
- *Toileting:* The ability to get on and off the toilet, bedpan or commode, and clean oneself after urinating and defecating.

Hygiene
The Nursing Assistant provides patient hygiene for those patients who are unable to cleanse themselves to:
- Keep weak patients comfortable and as odor-free as possible
- Reduce infections, irritations, and complications
- Reduce infestations by lice, fleas, and scabies mites

Bathing removes dead skin cells and oils that accumulate and cause irritation. Thoroughly cleanse, rinse and dry each area, as bacteria thrive in warm, dark and moist environments. Pay particular attention to skin care for the incontinent patient, as diarrhea is common in the end stages of many diseases, and enzymes in stools break down the skin. Carefully inspect your patient's skin, while maintaining privacy and modesty for your patient. Oral hygiene is important in this patient population, particularly for those with suppressed immune systems (e.g., AIDS patients), due to the risk of mucositis (inflammation of the lining of the mouth). Remove and cleanse dentures twice daily and check for breaks that irritate gums. Brush and floss the patient's own teeth twice daily.

Mobility
Encourage your patients to maintain or improve their mobility to increase their level of independence. Palliative and hospice patients rely on others for their care, so they risk becoming infantilized. Being able to transfer from the bed to a chair independently fosters their sense of accomplishment and allows the normal shifting of body tissues and fluids. Ensure your patients who need adaptive equipment for ambulation use it properly. When in doubt, arrange for a physiotherapist or occupational therapist to measure the canes, walkers and wheelchairs to be certain they provide maximum benefit and do not pose a safety threat. Reposition bedridden patients at least once every two hours, as it prevents fluids from accumulating in their lungs and digestive tracts, and relieves pressure on weight-bearing areas of the skin, such as the hips, shoulders and knees. The Nursing Assistant must report any

changes in mobility to the attending Registered Nurse.

Range of motion

Normal Range of Motion (ROM) occurs when your patient can move his or her joints through their natural, healthy arc, from flexion to extension. Physiotherapists and doctors measure ROM in degrees with a goniometer. *Active range of motion* is when your patient participates in the movement. *Passive range of motion* is when your patient does not participate in the movement. Patients with arthritis, edema, obesity, Lou Gehrig's disease (ALS), nerve damage, infections, postoperative surgical pain, and deformities have decreased Range of Motion.

Guide your patient through gentle, supportive ROM exercises to decrease joint limitations caused by disuse. Incorporate ROM exercises twice daily into your patient's bathing and dressing routines. To assist your patient with passive ROM, support the limb above and below the joint being exercised. Never force the joint into flexing or extending beyond its capability. Discontinue the motion immediately if the patient reports pain or show signs of pain, such as grimacing.

Range of Motion (ROM) exercises enable the joints of an immobile patient to move through their normal arc (extension and flexion). They include: Pelvic tilt; gastroc stretch; soleus stretch; single leg pull; table top; and hamstring stretch. It is the responsibility of the CNA to assist or perform these exercises with patients twice daily so that their muscles do not atrophy. ROM exercises are active or passive. In active ROM, the patient moves without assistance. In passive ROM, the patient is unable to move without assistance. When performing ROM, the CNA must provide support both above and below the joint being exercised, and move the joint gently and smoothly. Never force the joint to flex or extend beyond its capability, as pain and injury will result. If your patient is conscious and able to move, incorporate ROM exercises into routine ADL, such as dressing or bathing. Instruct family members in ROM exercises, if the patient and family so desire.

Nutrition

The Nursing Assistant may purchase food, prepare meals, and feed patients. Many end-stage patients report anorexia (lack of appetite) and changes in the taste of food from medications, disease, or treatments. Anorexia means decreased food consumption, problems meeting the patient's nutritional needs, and distress for the patient's family. *Total parenteral nutrition (TPN)* replaces all or some of the patient's food. TPN patients receive liquid nutrients through a surgically implanted feeding tube in the subclavian vein under the collarbone, or jugular vein of the neck, or umbilical vein in the abdomen, or PICC line in the arm. A 100 mL TPN bag is strapped around the ambulatory patient's waist or shoulder. Bedridden patients have a 500 mL — 4 L bag suspended from an IV pole. A battery-powered infusion pump delivers nutrients directly into the digestive system. TPN can cause discord in the family and ethical issues for caregivers because it prolongs life artificially. TPN removes the patient's pleasure and sense of normalcy from eating.

As death approaches, gastrointestinal (GI) function decreases, so your patients may experience constipation and abdominal distention. Constipation ranges from mild to severe and can require fecal disimpaction. Nausea and vomiting are often present, especially in end-stage patients with gynecological or gastrointestinal cancers, or AIDS. Nausea and vomiting causes anorexia (patients do not feel like eating or drinking). Even if they are hungry, they may avoid eating or drinking, due to the fear of returning nausea and vomiting. Anorexic patients quickly become dehydrated, malnourished, and lose stamina. They can develop fatal electrolyte imbalances that cause cardiac arrest. Depressed patients may refrain from eating because they want to die sooner. Family members often become angry with the patient for what they view as surrendering to the disease. Criticism about eating causes emotional distress for your patient and his or her direct caregivers. The CNA supports the patient through this difficult time by giving empathy, adjusting food, and notifying the dietician and nurse.

Near the end of life, nutritional needs change dramatically, and food may become more of a comfort than a necessity. Slowing of the gastrointestinal tract means many foods that the patient once enjoyed may now cause gastrointestinal discomfort, such as abdominal pain, nausea, vomiting, diarrhea, constipation, or bleeding. Many end-stage patients have a diminished sense of taste, or taste is altered as a result of medication, surgery or age. The mechanics of chewing (mastication) and swallowing (deglutition) become impaired, so that they are unable to eat normally or without significant assistance. Be aware of the cultural aspects of food. Recognize that some cultures have beliefs about specific food having healing qualities or soothing aspects. Respect these multicultural beliefs and values. If you are concerned regarding your patient's cultural beliefs about food, seek information from the dietician, chaplain, or your hospital library. Ask the nurse to check your institution's policy regarding multicultural foods.

Allow your patient to share meals with other patients, if he or she so desires. It is helpful to schedule meals around the timing of analgesic medication if pain is an issue. Provide personal care prior to eating, so your patient will be comfortable. However, take care not to tire your patient prior to eating. If your patient is able, encourage him or her to get out of bed, as the transfer to the chair and the upright position will aid digestion. Ask your patient for his or her meal preferences. If your patient has family or friends to eat with, schedule meals so they can be present. Keep in mind that many patients will require multiple small meals per day. Also remember that eating takes energy. Be considerate if your patient uses feeding tubes; do not have food or the aroma of food around your patient, which will make him or her feel deprived.

Grooming

A well-groomed appearance helps the Palliative Care and Hospice patient and his or her family cope with the health condition. Ensure your patients who wear eyeglasses, dentures or hearing aids have them in place while awake, to help them remain oriented to their surroundings. However, if a patient chooses not to wear aids, respect those wishes. The Nursing Assistant must respect the wishes of the patient and family regarding clothing choices and accessories (e.g., hair ribbons, make-up, and nail polish), especially religious clothing (e.g., yarmulke, hijab, sindoor, and turbans). Be aware of the fit of your patient's clothing. Ensure clothing does not bind, pinch, or restrict your patient's movement, and that no folds or creases are present that may cause skin breakdown. If your patient must wear a Johnny gown for examinations or incontinence, then protect your patient's modesty by tying one gown at the back, and one at the front, so your patient's rump is not exposed.

As patients approach death, they are often unable to clear debris, secretions and mucus accumulated in the mouth. Use oral suction swabs with sodium bicarbonate and peroxide to clear the accumulation and comfort your patient. Many patients are mouth-breathers which causes significant drying of the mucus membranes and tongue, so use a protective gel, like Oralbalance, and a humidifier to ease the discomfort associated with this dryness. If your patient wears dentures, remove them from the mouth and clean them at least twice daily. Assist your conscious patient with cleansing his or her own dentures to promote independence. Follow your institution's policy and procedure for denture care if your patient is unable to cleanse the dentures independently. Inspect your patient's mouth during oral care. Report sores, lesions, obstructions, or discolorations to the Registered Nurse.

For many patients nearing the end of life, there can be changes in their appearance that are difficult to face, one of which is related to their hair. Hair may be brittle, dry or fall out as a result of medications, disease or aging. Clean hair, styled in the patient's choice (or family's choice if the patient is unconscious) is important. Cleanse your patient's hair with gentle massage to detect pressure ulcers on the scalp. If your patient uses oxygen tubing or glasses, visually inspect the skin around the ears. There are commercial devices available that allow shampooing to be performed while the patient is in bed (e.g., EZ-Shampoo inflatable sink). Cleanse your patients' hands and feet and trim or file nails to avoid scratches. Pay particular attention to the feet of the bedridden patient, as heels are a common area for pressure ulcers.

Almost all Hospice and Palliative Care patients will eventually require assistance in performing their activities of daily living (ADL). ADL includes preparation, execution, and clean up for bathing, eating, mobility and toileting. Personal care of the patient includes: Inspection of the skin for signs of irritation or breakdown: monitoring of food and liquid intake and output; positioning the patient with good body alignment and support; dressing the patient, including any appliances, such as hearing aids and/or glasses. Personal care is an ongoing process and because many end-stage patients experience pain and fatigue, it is important that the CNA schedule the performance of personal care at times that stress the patient the least. Incontinence care should be performed when necessary, but always with the patient's comfort in mind. It is the responsibility of the CNA to provide privacy for the patient while performing personal care.

Toileting

The Nursing Assistant must report any changes in the patient's bladder and bowel habits to the Registered Nurse, as these may be a result of medication, diet, and/or disease processes. Your patient may need toilet adaptive equipment, such as a raised toilet seat or railings. The Nursing Assistant must provide urinary catheter care for patients who have indwelling Foley catheters, to prevent urinary tract infections. Catheter care is best conducted while the patient is reclined (supine). Report any change in catheter output, and foul-smelling, bloody, cloudy, or smoky urine to the Registered Nurse, because it could indicate kidney damage. The Nursing Assistant cares for ostomy patients by becoming familiar with the different ostomy products, and conducting careful inspection of the skin surrounding the stoma with each change of apparatus. Report any change in fecal output or skin appearance to the Registered Nurse.

Difficulties with incontinence care: heavy lifting, psychological trauma, social stigma, timely hygiene and odor and infection control.

Steps for incontinence care:
1. Bring patient to private area immediately after soiling
2. Don gloves; protect area with sheet
3. Position patient lateral, supine, or squatting
4. Remove and bag soiled clothing
5. Wipe perineum and contaminated skin with:
6. Mild soap on wet washcloth and rinse with warm water OR
7. No-rinse perineal wash and cotton
8. Dry with a soft cloth
9. Inspect perineum for infection (redness, blisters, or discharge)
10. Apply silicone barrier cream to reduce skin breakdown
11. Apply clean incontinence product; adjust clothing and patient position
12. Report changes in frequency, color, and consistency of excreta to the RN

Products:

Bowel and bladder training: Bowel and bladder training regimes are usually used to train patients who have a chance of recovery for eventual continence, for example, after pelvic surgery. Hospice and Palliative Care patients are end-stage, so the goal of this training is patient comfort. It is the responsibility of the CNA to work with the interdisciplinary team, patient and family to understand and implement a bowel or bladder regime or training program. When a program is already in place, the CNA investigates if the plan is working for the patient and his or her family. The CNA must follow the program as delineated, without deviation. However, if the CNA suspects that the program is unsatisfactory for the patient or family, the CNA reports the problem to the Registered Nurse, so an alternative plan can be developed. The CNA is an important member of the interdisciplinary team and should have input into the development of a plan.

Comparison of Incontinence Products		
	Disposable	*Reusable*
Pros	Harder to tear off, so they are suitable for confused or infected patients	Cheaper More environmentally friendly
Cons	Expensive	Difficult to store for laundering
After Soiling	If your patient is *infection-free*, disposable products are Group E; place them in household garbage. If your patient is *infected*, disposable products are Group A; put them in a yellow biohazard bag for incineration, or autoclaving and shredding.	Conscientiously separate reusable pads for laundering. Mixing pads from different patients or with other clothes spreads disease.

Enemas:

ENEMAS	
Definition: Irrigating the bowel	
Purpose: Bowel cleansing; barium x-ray; constipation relief; decrease abdominal distention; relieve gas pain and pressure; feed anorexics; lower fever	
Ordered By: Physician only, because enemas may interfere with fluid balance	
Administered By: • CNA gives saline, oil, or phosphate (Fleet) enemas • RN gives medicated enema in case of adverse drug reaction • Radiographer gives barium enema for x-ray of your patient's lower GI tract	Safe fluid amounts: • Adult 750 cc—1 liter • School-aged child 500 cc—1 liter • Toddler less than 500 cc • Infant less than 250 cc

Equipment:
- Disposable enema (e.g., Fleet, Ped Fleet) *OR* 4 quart enema bag with clamp; 20—22 CH catheter, or 22—24 French Foley catheter with 30 cc balloon; 20 cc syringe; Toilet, commode, bedpan, or 2 gallon container; Thermometer
- K-Y jelly or water-soluble lubricant; Privacy curtain
- Odor control product; Hook to hold bag
- If bottled saline is unavailable, mix exactly 1 liter tap water with 1½ teaspoons of table salt for saline enema

Procedure:
- Ensure patient has no contraindications (e.g., rectal bleeding, appendicitis, electrolyte or fluid imbalance, etc.)
- Draw curtain or close door; Remove patient's pants
- Place patient lying on left side in Sim's position, if possible
- Lubricate patient's anus; Test enema solution with thermometer; it should be no warmer than 105°F to lessen cramping

- Insert catheter gently into rectum; do not force
- Instill fluid slowly to avoid pain from sudden pressure; the higher the bag, the faster the flow
- Gently hold buttocks together to retain fluid 5 min., if possible
- Seat patient on toilet for 30 min.

Timing and odor control

The CNA must time routine care appropriately. If your patient is unconscious, determine the schedule with the family. If your patient is conscious and coherent, let him or her determine the schedule as much as possible. Perform incontinence care immediately whenever the patient soils (PRN). Before performing personal care for an unconscious, visually impaired, or hearing impaired patient, identify yourself and explain what tasks you will perform. Encourage the family to participate in the patient's care, but respect the wishes of the patient and family. People are sensitive to odors, so keep your patient clean and as odor free as possible. If odors from incontinence and cancer are difficult to eliminate, try putting a tray of clean kitty litter or charcoal under your patient's bed to absorb odors.

Odor control for the Hospice and Palliative Care patient is important and often difficult, as many patients become incontinent and odors from diseases, wounds and ostomies are unpleasant. Keep your patient as clean as possible, and use some of the many commercially available products that cover or neutralize odors. When performing your patient's personal hygiene routine, especially incontinence care or bathing, control your facial expression and do not visibly react to unpleasant odors. If possible, perform hygiene tasks prior to the arrival of visitors. If family and friends are present, your patient's privacy is your primary concern. Ask your conscious patient about his or her preference regarding the presence of visitors during personal care. Ask visitors to leave while you perform care on the unconscious patient. When possible, give personal care in the bathroom with the door closed.

Scheduling tasks

When providing care for the dying patient, it is important that your timing coincides with the needs of the patient and family. Your patient will experience significant fatigue and requires increased sleep near the end of life, so work with the patient and family to determine the best time to provide personal care. Encourage family members to participate in the care of the patient, providing he or she agrees. Schedule care for times when pain medication is at its peak, so care does not cause significant pain. Incontinence care must be provided when necessary, as soon as the patient soils. Complete your patient's personal care in such a way that maximizes the time the patient spends awake with family and loved ones.

Maintaining patient independence

Aging, surgery and disease take a toll on patients because they lose independence and mobility. The role of the CNA is to foster independence in the patient according to his or her capability. Although it is faster and more convenient for the CNA to perform activities for the patient, it is psychologically more important for the patient to do as much as he or she desires to maintain a sense of independence and accomplishment. Cultural influences will impact the patient's independence. It is the CNA's responsibility to understand and respect the culture of each patient. For ambulatory patients, schedule periods of activity around pain medication and meals, to decrease fatigue.

Clothing

Many patients experience significant changes in their appearance through disease, surgery, aging or a combination of these, so appearance can be very important to them. Patients may be angry that they can no longer care for themselves. Patients may derive great pleasure from having control of the simple choice of what to wear. Although the CNA may disagree, it is up to the patient and his or her family to decide. It is the CNA's responsibility to ensure clothing fits properly, has no folds or creases that may lead to a pressure ulcer, or restrictive bands that inhibit breathing or cause pain. Clothes should be clean, in good condition, and odor-free. Some patients have favorite items of clothing and should be allowed to wear these as often as they like.

Hearing aids and glasses

Your patient has the right to choose whether to wear or remove his or her hearing aids or glasses. Respect your patient's wishes. If your patient chooses not to wear glasses, ensure there is sufficient light in the room to enhance vision. When your patient is not wearing eyeglasses or a hearing aid, ensure that the patient knows all who are present and what they are doing in the room. Encourage communication with any patient who has a visual or hearing deficit. Encourage families to keep the patient involved. When hearing aids and glasses are worn, inspect the skin on your patient's nose and ears to ensure no pressure ulcers are developing. Keep hearing aids and glasses within your patient's reach, clean and ready for use by the patient who does not require assistance with them.

Positioning

Immobile patients

The CNA must change the position of an immobile patient to avoid pressure ulcers and pneumonia, and promote fluid drainage. 30% of patients with one amputated limb need the limb on the opposite side amputated within five years because of poor circulation. Reposition an unconscious patient at least once every two hours. Reposition a conscious patient as frequently as requested. Maintain proper anatomical alignment when possible. Use padding, pillows and cushions to support and protect bony areas, and elevate edematous limbs. Do not allow folds or creases in clothing or bed sheets because they promote bedsores. Choose jersey knit sheets when possible, as they are better tolerated by bedridden and incontinent patients. Lung fluids pool in immobile patients; changing positions shifts the fluid to ease breathing. Carefully inspect the skin during bathing and repositioning. Report any red or open areas to the Registered Nurse. Position the patient to relieve pressure from any areas that appear at risk for the development of pressure ulcers.

The CNA is responsible for positioning patients who are immobile or uncoordinated to avoid bedsores and contractures. Your patient's medical condition may make certain positions more comfortable and beneficial than others. Avoid placing a patient with breathing difficulty (dyspnea) in the supine position (reclining on the back). Instead, use the semi-Fowler or orthopneic (upright and leaning forward) positions to allow easy respiration. A left side-lying position (Sim's) often proves beneficial for the patient with abdominal distension or ascites. Changing positions gently and carefully is important for the comfort of your patient. Use supports to maintain proper body alignment. Schedule the repositioning to coincide with the peak effectiveness of pain medication, but at a minimum of every two hours. Smooth creases and folds out of bed sheets and clothing because they can lead to pressure ulcers.

Patient transfers
Safety is paramount during a patient transfer. Prior to the transfer, plan the move with your patient. Have all necessary equipment nearby and ready to use. Get an assistant or use a hoist if your patient is heavy. Each person involved should know his or her role, and in which direction the patient will be moved. If your patient is capable of assisting with the transfer, ask him or her to grab the side rails of the bed and sit up. Lock wheelchair brakes to prevent rolling. Ideally, use a stand-pivot transfer, where your patient grabs the front of the wheelchair, and you brace him or her during the turn and sit. Use a board as a bridge between the bed and the wheelchair if your patient cannot stand. If your stroke patient has one weak side, always transfer toward the strong side. Use proper body mechanics to prevent injury. Instruct the patient's family members, if they so desire, in the proper way to perform transfers.

Adaptive equipment
Hospice and Palliative Care patients commonly need adaptive equipment. The responsibilities of the Nursing Assistant are to understand the equipment, use it properly, and teach the patient and family members how to use the equipment

properly. Commonly used adaptive equipment includes: Wheelchairs; walkers; canes; slide boards; Hoyer lifts; cushions; and pumps. Adaptive equipment is designed to make ADL easier for the patient and to decrease the physical burden placed on caregivers. Many devices require careful measurement and individual fitting by a physiotherapist, prosthetist, or occupational therapist. As patients gain or lose weight, it is important the devices they are using continue to function within their scope. Cushions for wheelchairs and beds are of particular importance for those patients who are unable to change position independently, because folds or creases can lead to skin breakdown.

Safety issues
A primary responsibility of the CNA is patient safety. If your patient is ambulatory, ensure the environment is free from hazards, such as scatter rugs that may cause the patient to slip. Ensure the patient has appropriate footwear to prevent slips and falls. Install a night-light. Do not be reluctant to turn on lights during the night to assist your patient, as adequate lighting can prevent a serious fall. Safety also includes: Proper use of adaptive equipment; good body mechanics when assisting with transfers; and protecting the integrity of the skin. Careful inspection of the skin when performing personal care, being certain bed sheets are smooth and wrinkle-free, and that the patient is positioned with proper body alignment are all safety measures for the patient.

Pressure ulcers

Definition	Pressure ulcers are preventable bedsores, also called decubitus ulcers, which indicate neglect and poor nursing care. A pressure ulcer can develop in as little as 8 hours.
At-Risk Patients	Bedridden, paralyzed, and terminal patients who are unable to change position independently
Mechanisms	<ul><li>Pressure on weight-bearing areas for an extended time period</li><li>Friction from casts, sheets, and braces</li><li>Prolonged cold exposure</li></ul>
Results	1. Blood circulation is cut off 2. Skin breakdown occurs 3. Painful tissue damage and necrosis (tissue death) develop
Areas Affected	Bony prominences, e.g., tailbone (coccyx), hips, knees, heels, elbows, and shoulders

Stages of skin damage and treatment:
- Stage I: Redness; disappears a few hours after pressure is relieved
- Stage II: Blistering; use moisturizer bandages
- Stage III: Wound extends through all skin layers (crater); antibiotics, duoderm, silvadene
- Stage IV: Blackening (eschar) extends through muscle, tendons and bone; debridement physiotherapy surgery
- Stage V: Wound extends to internal organs; amputation

Change your patient's position frequently, at least every two hours and use padding and cushions. Ensure adequate hygiene and nutrition (vitamin C, protein and fluids) and notify the registered nurse.

Stage 1

Stage 1 of a pressure ulcer is the appearance of reddened skin, usually over a bony prominence such as the hips, shoulders, knees, heels, buttocks, or elbows. In a person with darkly pigmented skin, the area may appear lighter in color. This area of redness or lightened color does not return to its normal color when the patient is repositioned and the pressure is relieved. If you discover a Stage 1 pressure ulcer, immediately reposition the patient so that pressure is relieved and reposition at least every 2 hours to prevent the ulcer from worsening. Do not massage the irritated skin or aggressively scrub it during bathing. Take care when positioning the patient to avoid friction and shearing injuries, particularly if your patient has thin "steroid skin". The skin must be kept clean and dry, particularly in folds, where skin touches skin. Use pillows, padding, and blankets to help position and support the patient.

Stage 2

A Stage 2 pressure ulcer has advanced to blistered, cracked or peeling skin. Skin is the first line of defense against infection, so a Stage 2 pressure ulcer puts the patient at risk for serious bacterial infections, like Pseudomonas and ßeta hemolytic Streptococci. Stay alert for warmth, foul odor, swelling, increasing pain, and pus, as these are signs of infection. Pay careful attention to hygiene, particularly for incontinent patients. Reposition the patient frequently to avoid applying pressure to the area. Take great care to avoid additional shearing or friction injuries to the area. Cushions are helpful in positioning the patient, but avoid inflatable doughnut rings, because they can decrease circulation further.

Check the patient's care plan to find out which moisturizing products you should use on the skin after bathing.

Stage 3

A Stage 3 pressure ulcer occurs when all layers of skin have eroded away and the underlying tissue is exposed in a *crater*. The deep tissue is damaged and there may be drainage from the wound. Although the damage is extensive, Stage 3 patients may not report pain if there damage to the nerves in the area (*neuropathy*). Excellent hygiene is necessary for the Stage 3 patient, because the risk for infection is very high. Bacteremia will develop in 4% of patients. MRSA (methicillin-resistant Staphylococcus aureus) develops in 30% of patients, and VRE (Vancomycin-resistant enterococci) is becoming more common. The doctor may not order antibiotics, to reduce the chance of developing deadly antibiotic-resistant strains of bacteria. Silvadene reduces bacteria. Position the patient on a specialized air mattress so no pressure is exerted on the ulcer site. Inspect the area frequently for signs of pocketing (tunneling under the skin). Skin may bleed with the slightest pressure from a swab, so use Duoderm. White tissue in the wound indicates *malignancy* (cancer).

Stage 4

A Stage 4 pressure ulcer has exposed bone and joints. The wound has *eschar* (black tissue) that is *necrotic* (dead). The patient may have *osteomyelitis* (bone infection) that requires amputation. Your institution may term this Stage 4 or Stage 5, but the latter term is being phased out. Stage 4 pressure ulcers have drainage present and the patient is at extreme risk for infection. The physician may order bed cradles, heel protectors, a specialty mattress, medication, nutritional support, and flap reconstruction surgery. Follow the care plan exactly and report any changes in the wound to the Registered Nurse. Turn the patient frequently, but use extreme care when repositioning to avoid friction and shearing. Keep the skin clean, dry, and hygienic.

Skin breakdown

One of the major problems for the immobile patient is the development of skin breakdown. Since the skin is the first line of defense against infection, it is imperative that it remains intact. Given the disease, nutritional and immobility states of these patients, careful inspection and intervention are vital for assuring patient safety. It is the responsibility of the CNA to visually inspect the patient's skin under adequate light during personal care, repositioning at every opportunity. The first sign of skin breakdown is the appearance of reddened areas of skin that are warm to the touch. If the patient has darkly pigmented skin, then the area may appear lighter, rather than reddened. Skin breakdown is most common over bony prominences, such as the shoulders, hips, knees, heels, and elbows. Repositioning at least once every two hours to keep the patient's full weight off these sites reduces the chance of bedsores. Report any skin breakdown to the Registered Nurse.

As people age, the upper layers of skin (*epidermis*) become thinner, and the fatty *subcutaneous tissue* that sits just under the skin decreases. The blood supply to the skin and subcutaneous tissue decreases, which makes the skin more fragile. Tissue loss and blood supply decrease mean the skin's ability to regenerate and heal is diminished. Even gentle pressure applied to elderly skin may result in an injury, especially if the patient has been taking steroids for a long time. The most common hospice injury is a skin tear, where the upper epidermis is torn from the underlying subcutaneous tissue. Any break in the skin increases the possibility of infection and should be cared for immediately and appropriately. Take great care when moving elderly patients because of the fragility of their skin. The CNA should not wear rings with prong settings or high-set stones, or other sharp jewelry that may inadvertently scratch the patient.

Environment issues

Most Palliative Care and Hospice patients, whether in their own home or an inpatient facility, prefer to have personal objects with them in their rooms as they approach death. It is important that the CNA understands the cultural and religious significance of these objects and treats all the patient's possessions with respect and care. It is easy for the home environment of the hospice patient to be transformed into a medical setting through the presence of medical equipment, medications, and even a hospital bed. If the CNA makes the room look more like a home bedroom than a hospital room, then it is less psychologically stressful for the patient and visitors. Add personal items for viewing. Store medical equipment in a closet or out of sight. Keep the patient's environment clean, orderly, sweet smelling and free of hazards.

Just as healthy individuals appreciate a change in scenery, so do confined patients. When possible, assist the patient to move to other environments. Distract and relax the patient with a different view, preferably a nature view in fresh air. When assisting the patient with moving from one environment to another, remember that end-stage patients are easily fatigued and cannot control body temperature well. Explain to the family that simply going outside for a few minutes can prove to be exhausting for the patient, even if he or she does not complain. It is important to include the family and caregivers in this activity if the patient so desires. Be attentive to the patient and allow him or her to determine when to return to the sick room.

As patients approach death, they experience many psychological changes that accompany the physiologic changes that result from disease and/or aging. The emotional energy a patient must exert to come to terms with impending death is exhausting. Many patients may not show outward signs of this energy expenditure, but they are struggling with how to say good-bye to everything they know and care about. Keep the patient's environment calm to assist the patient, family and caregivers with managing emotion as they struggle with loss. Maintain order and cleanliness in the immediate living area of the patient. Have items requested by the patient within easy reach or within view. Keep the lighting level as most preferred by the patient to promote relaxation and comfort.

The CNA must provide the patient in a residential facility with most comfortable, homelike environment possible to decrease stress. If the patient is homebound, then minimize the appearance of clinical apparatus; cover it when it is not in use. Encourage the family to bring in items from the patient's home that may offer comfort. Make religious or culturally significant articles available. Treat all items that belong to the patient with the utmost respect and keep them safe. While understanding and respecting the patient's cultural beliefs is important in providing care to the patient and family, agreement is unnecessary.

Care location choice

Patients have the right to die in their places of choice, if at all possible. Advanced medical care may require moving the patient to hospital, but make every effort to honor the patient's wishes regarding where he or she wants to die. Anticipate disagreement within the patient's family regarding the patient's choice. Acknowledge cultural issues that may play a role in their decision. Reassure patients and families that their choices need not be based on cultural expectations, but on what is best for them. The most important aspect is that their choice truly is the desire of the patient and family, and not the result of outside influences.

Circulatory system

Vital signs include temperature, pulse, respiratory rate and blood pressure and are reported in that order. As a patient nears death, the circulatory system slows and is unable to deliver blood effectively. Poor peripheral circulation means blood is shunted away from the extremities and delivered to the vital organs (heart, kidneys, and brain), which elevates the patient's core temperature up to 104°F (40°C). The rise in temperature stimulates perspiration in an effort to normalize the body's temperature to

98.6°F (37°C). The combination of decreased circulation in the extremities and increased perspiration causes the patient to feel cool and clammy to the touch. Although your patient's body may feel cool, use only light bed coverings, as the core is actually hot. Heavy blankets may cause your patient discomfort, which leads to restlessness. Explain this process to your patient's family, so they are not concerned that their loved one is receiving inappropriate care.

Respiratory issues

Breathing exercises
More than 50% of dying patients experience dyspnea at some time during the process of dying, so the CNA must encourage and work with the patient to perform breathing exercises that can help alleviate dyspnea. Your patient must inhale air deeply into the lungs to oxygenate the tissues. These factors decrease the depth of inhalation and prevent adequate oxygenation: Pain; respiratory disease (e.g., emphysema, asthma, cystic fibrosis, and asbestosis); ascites; arthritic ribs; wear and tear from aging; and increased mucus accumulation in the respiratory tract. Deep breathing and coughing exercises move mucus out of the lungs, bronchi, pharynx, and nasal mucosa, allowing more oxygen to be absorbed. Place the patient in semi-Fowler's, Fowler's or the orthopneic position to assist with breathing. Use incentive spirometry per doctor's order, and document the number of times per day and the settings in the patient's care plan. Many patients report a decrease in dyspnea with the use of fans, but this should not be considered a replacement for breathing exercises.

Oxygen administration
Oxygen is classified as a medication and as such each state determines under the Registered Nurse Practice Act just what a CNA can and cannot do when caring for patients with oxygen. The CNA is required to be familiar with state laws regarding oxygen administration, and to be properly trained in administering oxygen if the state permits it. The CNA must know the oxygen flow rate the physician has ordered for the patient, and report to the Registered Nurse any time the flow rate does not agree with the order. Oxygen can be administered through nasal cannulae (prongs at the end of tubing), masks, or blow-by technique if the patient resists the mask. Inspect the patient's skin under the cannulae and cleanse it twice daily. Ensure the tubing is not kinked or twisted, which hampers the oxygen flow. Follow the safety rules surrounding oxygen at all times. Do not allow your patient or visitors to smoke in the presence of oxygen.

Reportable breathing patterns
Report these changes in breathing patterns to the Registered Nurse:
- *Tachypnea:* Fast respiratory rate greater than 20 per minute, signaling pain or respiratory distress
- *Bradypnea:* Abnormally slow rate of breathing (less than 12 per minute at rest)
- *Hyperventilation:* Rapid, deep breathing from fear, exertion, or oxygen starvation, which results in dizziness and fainting
- *Hypoventilation:* Inadequate breathing or reduced lung function that allows carbon dioxide to increase in the blood

- *Dyspnea:* Difficulty in breathing or labored breathing
- *Paroxysmal nocturnal dyspnea (PND):* Sudden-onset dyspnea after going to sleep and awakening due to coughing, wheezing, tachycardia, and sweating. PND is a symptom of congestive heart failure (CHF), often caused by left ventricular failure and/or pulmonary edema.
- *Orthopnea:* Inability to breathe lying down. Patients with orthopnea sleep sitting up in a chair, or propped up in bed with pillows. Orthopnea is a symptom of congestive heart failure. Measure the severity of orthopnea by the number of pillows needed to prop up the patient in bed to permit breathing.

Respiratory failure

Patient's problem:
- Cannot clear mucus effectively
- Shortness of breath (SOB), dyspnea (difficulty breathing), and orthopnea (difficulty breathing except when sitting upright)
- Cheyne-Stokes breathing (Cycles of rapid, deep breathing, progressing to slow, shallow breathing, then apnea for 15—45 sec. Patient may awaken.)
- Death rattle wheezing when saliva and mucous collect in the upper airway as the palate relaxes. Loss of cough and swallow reflexes that clear the airway.
- Breathing stops, followed by 1—2 widely spaced breaths, then silence

CNA's duties:
- Clear patient's mouth with oral swabs
- Place patient in semi-Fowler or orthopneic position
- Elevate head of bed 30°—45°
- Change patient's position every 2 hours
- Notify RN at hospice, or doctor at home

RN's duties:
- Suctioning
- Inform doctor of Cheyne-Stokes
- Restrict fluids
- Pronounces death in hospice

Doctor's duties:
- Prescribes decongestants
- Prescribes opiates to ease breathing, but the patient may consequently develop myoclonic jerking
- Inform family death will occur
- Elevate head of bed 30°—45°
- If the family is distressed, prescribes:
  o Diphenhydramine (Benadryl) to dry secretions
  o Scopolamine patch behind ear every 3 days to block vagal reflex
  o One drop of 1% Atropine sublingually every 2 hours to decrease noise
  o Pronounces death anywhere

Dyspnea

Dyspnea is difficulty breathing; develops in 50-70% of dying patients. Associated most with: Lung or breast cancer; heart disease; pneumonia; emphysema; lung or heart tissue damage from radiation or chemotherapy; and diseases that cause fluid retention. However, any end-stage patient can develop dyspnea. Dyspnea is upsetting to the patient and family, as it is a form of suffering difficult to control. Even if your patient cannot speak, you can tell if your patient has dyspnea, because he or she:

- Uses accessory muscles to breathe (parasternal, scalene, sternocleidomastoid, trapezius, and pectoralis)
- Has distended neck veins from respiratory effort
- Flares the nostrils

To help relieve your patient's dyspnea:
- Change your patient's position to semi-Fowler or orthopneic
- Open the window or use a fan to encourage air movement through the room
- Lower the thermostat, because cool temperatures may help (but not cold)
- Inform the registered nurse or respiratory therapist that the patient appears to need oxygen

Increased secretions in the respiratory tract

Dying patients have increased amounts of mucus secreted by their respiratory system and have difficulty clearing these secretions. If your patient is conscious, encourage deep breathing, coughing, and use of an incentive spirometer to clear the airway. Removing mucous by these methods becomes more difficult as the patient becomes weaker and pain increases, so the RN must suction the patient. Patients who use a nasal cannula or facemask to deliver supplemental oxygen experience significant drying of the mucus membranes of the nose and mouth, while still experiencing increased secretions in their lungs. If your patient is unable to clear respirator secretions, call the RN or Respiratory Therapist for suctioning. Neck-breathing patients with a tracheostomy require frequent suctioning. Mucus collects in the upper respiratory tract when the palate relaxes and the patient loses the gag and swallowing reflexes. The wheezing that results is referred to as the death rattle. It is not painful for the patient, but the doctor treats it if it distresses the family.

Cardiac activity changes

As patients approach death, they experience changes in their circulatory system, which is driven by the heart. End-stage patients commonly experience episodes of irregular heartbeats (arrhythmia), although not all patients exhibit this sign. Arrhythmia may be sporadic or sustained. The patient's pulse may become rapid (tachycardia, >100 bpm when the patient is at rest) and difficult to detect in the wrist. If tachycardia occurs, palpate the carotid artery in the neck *on one side only*. Applying pressure on both sides slows the heartbeat. If you cannot feel a carotid pulse, use a stethoscope to detect heart activity. This can be particularly distressing for the family to observe, as it can be viewed as confirmation that death is imminent. The CNA must be familiar with the patient's baseline cardiac status, so any changes will be noted and reported to the Registered Nurse. Use a vital sign flow sheet to track this information at least once per shift.

Nausea and vomiting

Approximately 40% of terminally ill patients experience nausea and vomiting at some time as they are dying. These symptoms are most common in patients with breast, stomach or gynecological cancers and patients dying of AIDS. Medications, including many taken for pain, may also cause nausea and vomiting because they irritate the GI tract. Nausea is a *symptom* because it is self-reported by the patient. If the patient is non-verbal, nausea is undetectable. Vomiting is a *sign* because it can be observed by staff and family. If the cause of nausea or vomiting is unknown, keep track of the circumstances under which the symptom and sign appear, so interventions can be developed. Vomiting distresses the patient and makes the family feel helpless when they are unable to resolve it. Include the family in the treatment plan because they can tell you what has been successful in the past for treating nausea and vomiting in the patient.

- Organ failure
- Oxygen deprivation
- Pain
- Sepsis

Fatigue

Fatigue occurs in 80% of dying patients. Fatigue is a *symptom,* based on the patient's subjective report, and cannot be objectively measured. *Ask* your patient if he or she is tired. Many patients will not report fatigue spontaneously. Causes of fatigue are:

- Anemia
- Anorexia
- Blood loss
- Constipation
- Dehydration
- Depression
- Hypercalcemia
- Insomnia
- Medications (opioids, sedatives, antinauseants, & antihistamines)
- Nausea & vomiting

Managing fatigue

How CNA Manages Patient Fatigue	Doctor's Prescription for Fatigue	
1. 1. Allow patient to restrict visitors 2. 2. Breathing exercises 3. 3. Conserve energy with assistive devices 4. 4. Minimize fatiguing activities 5. 5. Report change fatigue level to RN 6. 6. Schedule activities for times when patient has more energy	*Class*	*Drug*
	Antianxiety	Valium (diazepam) Ativan (lorazepam)
	Antiemetic	Zofran (ondansetron) Reglan (metoclopramide)
	Appetite Stimulant	Megace (megestrol acetate) Marinol (dronabinal)
	Bronchodilator	Albuterol Theophylline
	Corticosteroid	Decadron (dexamethasone)
	CNS Stimulant	Ritalin (methylphenidate)
	Laxative	Senekot (senna)
	Opioid	Morphine
	Sedative	Haloperidol (for delirium)
	Stool Softener	Pericolace (docusate)

Pain

Definition	Pain is a warning sensation designed to protect the body. Pain can be acute or chronic. Pain is a *symptom*, meaning it is subjective, self-reported by the patient, and cannot be measured objectively. Pain is whatever your patient says it is.
Types	• Breakthrough pain overcomes round-the-clock analgesics, like morphine • Incident pain is from moving or coughing • Idiopathic pain has no known cause and lasts longer than incident pain • End of dose failure means pain starts before the next scheduled dose of analgesic
Signs	A *sign* is a reaction that can be objectively seen and measured. Stay alert for these objective signs of pain, particularly in non-verbal patients: • Facial grimacing • Moaning • Restlessness • Guarding the sore area • Increased pulse, respiration and blood pressure

Pain Contributors: Fatigue; inactivity; pessimism; stress; inadequate sleep; overexertion; unpleasant smells
Cultures that suppress pain: East Indians; North American Plains Indians; British; Irish; "Old Americans"
Cultures that express pain: Italian; Jewish; Puerto Rican
Religions that view pain as the Will of God: Catholics; Hindus; Muslims; Buddhists

Disease Process: Neuropathy and CIPA prevent patients from perceiving pain and regulating their body temperatures. Ensure these patients are safe from injury because they cannot feel when they are hurt, frozen, or burnt. Patients with amputations continue to have phantom pain because the pain pathways (nociceptors) keep transmitting the sensation even after the limb is removed.

Monitoring pain levels

Many patients experience altered levels of consciousness near the end of life, and are unable to communicate symptoms verbally. It is imperative that the CNA and family monitor the patient for signs of pain, such as: Moaning, restlessness, wincing, and grimacing. Pay particular attention when these signs occur, as the patient may require pain medication prior to movement or dressing changes. Avoid positions that you know aggravate the patient, if possible. The healthcare team may be more objective in their assessment of pain, and the family may be more perceptive of the patient's needs. The best approach is to use everyone's knowledge to interpret signs of pain the patient is unable to communicate verbally. If you suspect your patient is in pain, or notice changes in the patient's condition, report these to the Registered Nurse.

Non-pharmaceutical interventions

In order to alleviate pain, it is important for the CNA to understand the patient's concept of pain and the cultural context in which it was developed. Try non-pharmaceutical interventions that have been previously successful for your patient first. If your patient is unable to tell you what worked in the past, consult the family. Carefully position your patient every two hours. Ensure bed linens are free of wrinkles and creases. Using the bedpan, urinal or bathroom also has been shown to reduce pain in many patients. Gentle touch or massage by either the CNA or a family member may make the patient more comfortable. Encourage your patient to listen to soft music, and view favorite movies, TV shows, or family videos and photos to distract him or her

from pain. Report unrelieved pain to the registered nurse immediately.

Determining effectiveness of pain treatment

One of the predominant aspects of palliative and hospice care is the focus on pain control and it is the CNA's responsibility to be aware of and report changes in the patients' pain, either an increase in pain or the resolution of it. Even if the patient is able to communicate with family and caregivers, he or she may not accurately report pain for cultural reasons or so as not to bother people. It is important for the CNA to be alert to these non-verbal signs of pain: Facial grimaces (particularly with movement); moaning; increased heart and respiratory rates; and an increase in blood pressure; restlessness; unusually quiet demeanor; and avoiding movement of an extremity (guarding). The evaluation of the effectiveness of any treatment for pain, whether through medication or other intervention, should include the decrease in non-verbal signs. It is also important for the CNA to understand the patient's definition of pain and the cultural expectations to express or repress pain.

Recognizing side effects

Fear of pain is the most common fear associated with dying. Pain management is a primary focus of care for the Palliative and Hospice patient. The use of opioid medications is common and it is the role of the CNA to be aware of and on the lookout for side effects. The most common side effects of opioids are drowsiness, confusion, nausea and constipation. Some patients may resist medication because they may view their pain as punishment or may not want to be sedated. If your patient becomes confused after receiving pain medication, approach him or her calmly. Reassure both the patient and the family that this is a side effect that will pass. Bowel regimes should be developed to decrease constipation. Time medication with or without food per doctor's order to assist with nausea. Report any changes in pain to the Registered Nurse.

Changes in pain patterns
End-stage patients experience multiple physiological changes. Some changes are a direct result of the specific disease process, while others are universal and related to the approach of death. If your conscious patient has experienced a significant amount of pain throughout the course of the disease (e.g., pancreatic cancer), when he or she reports a marked decrease in pain, death is imminent. A decrease in pain relates to medication overload in the patient's circulatory system as the filtering ability of the kidneys and liver decreases. As death nears, endorphins are released as natural analgesics, and the patient perceives a decrease in pain. However, some patients experience a marked increase in pain from disease process. Report changes in pain pattern to the Registered Nurse, as the patient may need bronchodilators, benzodiazepines, steroids, and a nerve block to relieve pain that cannot be controlled by opiates alone.

Edema and ascites

Edema is the accumulation of fluid in the interstitial spaces between cells, which causes swelling. It is important for the CNA to balance fluids for the dying patient to reduce edema. Severe edema is painful and puts the patient at risk for skin breakdown, decreased mobility,

compromised circulation, and dyspnea (difficulty breathing). By positioning the patient correctly, the CNA increases comfort and reduces edema by returning fluids back into the circulatory system. Edematous extremities should never be in a dependent position (hanging downwards). Report all changes in edema to the Registered Nurse.

Ascites is the accumulation of peritoneal fluid in the abdominal cavity and is usually a result of liver disease or damage (cirrhosis or cancer). This fluid buildup distends the abdomen and can result in dyspnea. Many patients with ascites find the left side-lying position is the most comfortable (Sim's position). Remind your patient to urinate frequently. Keeping the bladder empty provides some relief from ascites' discomfort.

Xerostomia and stomatitis

End-stage patients sleep more, so one of their common complaints is *xerostomia* (dry mouth and lips). Causes of xerostomia include: Candida (thrush); dehydration from decreased food and fluid intake; drying medications (e.g., Benadryl and Lasix); increased mouth breathing; and kidney failure. Patients with defective kidneys develop *uremic stomatitis*, which starts as mouth burning and dryness, progresses to gray exudate, and leads to severely bleeding mouth ulcers. It is the role of the CNA to provide oral care as frequently as necessary to alleviate xerostomia for the patient. Perform oral care for the unconscious patient with the patient in a side-lying position to avoid aspiration. For the conscious patient, frequent use of a soft bristled toothbrush or oral swabs is recommended. Examples of products that assist with treatment of xerostomia are Toothettes, saliva substitute, Oralbalance, Chapstick, and cold humidifiers. If lemon and glycerin swabs increase dryness, try gargling with 1 tsp. salt in 8 oz. tap water. Remove dentures for cleaning at least twice daily.

Ostomy care

Care of the patient with an ostomy varies little for the palliative care and hospice patient from care of any patient with an ostomy. As the patient's metabolism changes from decreased intake of food and fluids, there will be a decrease in ostomy output. If the patient has not decreased his or her intake, report any decrease in output to the Registered Nurse because it could mean an obstruction. Ostomy patients are at risk of skin breakdown as a result of contact with gastric secretions, adhesive, and feces. Carefully cleanse and inspect the skin and the stoma at each bag change. Ensure the ostomy pouch does not become trapped beneath the patient's clothing, as it may interfere with normal elimination and be a source of discomfort. Common odor control products include: M9 drops; DevKo tablets; and Flat D disks.

Food preparation

The CNA and interdisciplinary team must access community resources for patients who do not have caregivers in their own homes to attend to the details of daily living. Contact the patient's social worker, who will know of agencies in your area that provide meals for a nominal fee. You may just need to call Meals on Wheels if the patient is able to eat a regular diet, but is unable to prepare food. You may actively participate in food preparation if

a special diet is required, or if the patient needs multiple small meals throughout the day, rather than three large meals. Consult the patient and consider his or her food preferences. Contact a nutritionist to determine the nutritional needs of the patient and consistency of the food, based on the patient's ability to chew and swallow.

Feeding tubes

Patients who are unable to process food normally as the result of surgery, paralysis, disease, chemotherapy, or radiation therapy receive their nutrition through a feeding tube in the gastrointestinal tract.

- A nasogastric (NG) tube is inserted by the Registered Nurse or physician through the patient's nose and advanced into the stomach.
- A nasointestinal tube is introduced into the patient's nose and advanced into the intestine.
- A gastrostomy tube is surgically inserted through the abdominal wall into the stomach.
- A PEG (percutaneous endoscopic gastrostomy) tube is inserted surgically through the abdominal wall with the assistance of an endoscope. The endoscope allows the surgeon to see down the esophagus and into the stomach as the PEG tube is sutured (stitched) in place. Feedings through these tubes are either continuous or intermittent, and the feeding is most often controlled by an electronic pump.

Nasogastric feeding tubes

Indwelling feeding tubes are a potential source of infection. It is the role of the CNA to cleanse and monitor feeding tubes to prevent infection. Nasogastric tubes often cause irritation that develops into pressure ulcers. Clean the nasal passages every 4 to 8 hours, or as directed on the care plan. Patients with feeding tubes are at risk for aspiration (inhaling food particles into the lungs). It is the responsibility of the CNA to monitor the patient's respiratory status. If your patient has a feeding tube, then keep the head of the bed elevated to at least 30° at all times. Avoid the left side-lying position during a feeding, as this position is not conducive to emptying of the stomach. Perform oral care at least twice daily for patients with feeding tubes.

PEG tubes

Care of the patient with a PEG tube is the same as for a patient with any feeding tube, with the addition of the care of the insertion site. The site should be inspected, cleansed, and have the dressing changed according to the care plan, but minimally every 8 hours. Report any indication of skin breakdown to the Registered Nurse. Patients with PEG tubes often have their feedings run continuously. Continuous feedings are controlled by pumps. It is the responsibility of the CNA to know the rate at which the feeding should be delivered. However, the CNA is not responsible for programming or changing the rate of the pump; those are the duties of the nutritionist and RN. Careful positioning of the patient is important to prevent aspiration, pressure ulcers related to tube placement and dislodging of the PEG tube. Inspect the tube for kinks or twists that may interfere with the flow of formula.

Positioning the patient

The gastrointestinal tract moves food along in waves, called *peristalsis.* The feeding tube can dislodge through peristalsis. The Registered Nurse will carefully assess tube placement prior to use. If the patient is at home, a family member may be taught to do this. Careful positioning of the patient with a feeding tube is important, as it is possible for the feeding tube to be pulled out during movement. It is the responsibility of the CNA to be aware of the location of feeding tubes during personal care, position changes, transfers and ambulation. Patients with feeding tubes should not be in a supine position while a feeding is running or within one hour of a feeding, as they are at risk for vomiting and/or aspiration. Avoid the left side-lying position during or immediately after feedings, as this position delays stomach emptying.

Aspiration

Aspiration is the inhaling of objects or food into the lungs. Patients who have feeding tubes are at risk for aspiration. It is the responsibility of the CNA to know the signs of aspiration and to take measures that will help avoid this complication. Avoid the supine position while feedings are running. Report all adverse changes to the Registered Nurse immediately.

Signs of aspiration: Conscious patients may complain of chest pain, feeling full, and may prefer to sit upright, leaning forward. Conscious and unconscious patients can demonstrate:

- Audible wheezing
- 'Wet' sounding or productive cough
- Increased respiratory rate

- Increased pulse
- Cyanosis (a bluish color in the fingernails and/or around the mouth)
- Decreased oxygen saturation measurement

Comfort measures

Feeding tubes often represent to patients and their families the loss of their normal lives because most cultures attach significant importance to the sharing of food together. The patient's inability share a meal separates him or her from the family. Remind family members and caregivers to refrain from eating in the presence of the patient and to avoid wafting the aroma of food, as it reminds the patient of loss. Whether the patient has a PEG or a nasogastric tube, the insertion site must be monitored for skin breakdown. Cushions that protect the skin include SUR-FIT stomahesive and DURAHESIVE flat skin barrier. Adhesives include Skin-Tac H or Torbot Liquid Bonding Cement. Nasogastric tubes may cause the patient to feel choking or dyspnea. Secure the tube to the nose with special tape (e.g., Durapore Multi-purpose Silk-like surgical tape) to make the patient feel more secure.

IV therapy

Intravenous (IV) therapy is the delivery of fluids, medication, blood, nutrients, or a combination of these through a vein. The CNA does not administer an IV. IV therapy is delivered by a Registered Nurse. The role of the CNA is to observe the insertion site for signs of infection, ensure the IV tubing does not become kinked or twisted during patient movements, and ensure the IV catheter does not dislodge. Most IV solutions are administered through an IV infusion pump (e.g., Alaris, Baxter, and Sabratek). The rate of infusion is determined by the physician's order and the Registered Nurse is responsible for maintaining the accuracy of the settings on the pump. Call the RN if the pump alarms. IV therapy can be viewed by the family as a barrier between them and the patient, so make the family comfortable with its presence.

Central venous catheters

Central venous catheters (central lines) are used to monitor heart pressure and output, vascular resistance, and to deliver fluids when the patient's arms are not suitable for repeated IV punctures. Central lines are inserted by a physician under local anesthesia. The doctor makes a surgical opening in the arm or chest wall, advances the tube into a major vessel (e.g., subclavian or internal jugular), and into the vena cava on the right side of the heart. Central lines have more potential for serious complications than peripheral IV lines. Patients with central lines can develop: *Pneumothorax* (air in the chest that collapses the lung); *hemothorax* (bleeding in the chest); stroke if the tubing disconnects; *hematoma* (severe bruising); and infection. Care for a central line as you would a peripheral line.

Peripheral Intravenous (IV) therapy

A peripheral IV is usually inserted by an Emergency Medical Technician or Registered Nurse into a vein in the patient's arm or back of the hand. In babies, veins in the scalp and feet are often used. Inspect IV sites for redness, swelling, heat and drainage. Complications of IV therapy are:
- Infection (septicemia and cellulitis)

- Infiltration (IV fluid leaks through the walls of the vein, and enters the interstitial spaces in the arm tissues, rather than the vein)
- Blood clots
- Phlebitis
- Fluid overload (distended neck veins, increased blood pressure, and respiratory distress)

Report changes in the appearance of the IV site to the Registered Nurse.

Mental and emotional issues

End-stage patients experience multiple emotional changes with multifaceted causes. Cultural beliefs surrounding death may be responsible, as many cultures approach death as a fearful subject and experience. Religious beliefs may lead some patients to view illness and impending death as punishment for accomplishments or failures in their lifetime. Even those patients at peace with the approach of their death report emotional changes, ranging from anger directed at themselves, their family, and/or God, to calm and a sense of great peace. Much of the emotional response of the patient is related to the cultural and spiritual beliefs of the patient and family. Be aware of these beliefs and be supportive of the patient and their family.

Metabolic changes result when the patient decreases caloric intake and becomes dehydrated. Mild dehydration releases *endorphins* that relieve pain and produce *euphoria* (a sense of well-being). Kidney failure causes nitrogenous waste products (urea and creatinine) to build up in the blood (*azotemia*) and your patient will become confused. Liver failure causes *hepatic encephalopathy*, where the patient

is confused, then stuporous, and slips into coma. The physician determines whether or not to investigate the causes of kidney and liver failure, as the tests cause discomfort and the metabolic imbalance may not be treatable. Changes in mental status may also be related to *hypoxia* (lack of oxygen), medications or delirium. Delirium can be caused by an infection. Some patients develop *terminal restlessness* in the day or two prior to death. Restlessness may also be caused by urinary retention, constipation and pain. Observe the patient carefully to determine the cause and subsequent treatment. Support and reassure the family, who will be distressed at seeing mental changes in their loved one.

Confusion
It is not uncommon for the Palliative Care and Hospice patient to experience episodes of confusion. Depending on the underlying disease process, these episodes may be short-lived or grow progressively more frequent and long lasting. Possible causes of confusion, beginning with the most common, are: Changes in medications; decreased metabolizing of medications; decreased respiratory function resulting in hypoxia; altered sleep patterns; anxiety; pain; urinary retention; constipation; kidney and liver failure; sepsis; and terminal restlessness. Carefully observe the patient to determine the cause of confusion. Keep the room calm, clean, and orderly. Support the patient and educate the family to expect confusion from metabolic changes.

Level of responsiveness
As patients approach death, they experience metabolic changes from the disease process, kidney and liver failure,

dehydration, and a significant decrease in nutrients. These metabolic changes decrease the patient's level of responsiveness. Other reasons for decreased responsiveness include: Pain control medications; significant fatigue; psychological withdrawal; hypoxia (decreased ability to absorb oxygen); or changes in blood sugar (hypoglycemia or hyperglycemia). The doctor may choose not to investigate the cause of changes in the level of responsiveness extensively, as the tests are invasive and cause discomfort to the patient. Educate the patient's family to expect a decreased level of responsiveness. Support the patient who desires quiet and calm during this time.

Determining effectiveness of interventions

The CNA performs many interventions that are beneficial to the patient and family. The CNA explores the patient's cultural and religious beliefs to help him or her express fear and anxiety. It is the responsibility of the CNA to monitor the patient for these signs of the effectiveness of interventions:

- Decreased anxiety
- Increased calmness
- Decreased restlessness and agitation
- Increased ability to talk with family and loved ones
- Decreased complaints of pain
- An overall improvement in the patient's interactions with the world
- Less frequent use of analgesics and self-administered pain pump

Many patients experience a sense of isolation. Increased interaction with family and caregivers is significant, as it indicates a change in focus from the patient and the dying process to activities outside the patient.

Functional changes

End-stage patients decrease their food and liquid intake. Less caloric energy is available for activity. They often experience *vital exhaustion (VE),* marked by severe fatigue, weakness, irritability, and demoralization. VE often starts a few weeks before a heart attack (MI) and sudden cardiac death, especially in women and the elderly. Depression and insomnia often overlap with VE. Functional abilities and mobility decline because of the fatigue, so the patient requires increasing assistance from the CNA, family and caregivers. Schedule care so the patient has the most energy when family and friends are visiting. Use caution when assisting fatigued patients to ambulate, as a fatigued patient is at a greater risk for falling. Educate the family to expect decreased function and mobility and increased dependency.

The most common symptom reported by end-stage patients is fatigue, often accompanied by weakness (vital exhaustion). *Vital exhaustion* is a strong predictor that the patient is stressed and will have a cardiac episode. The adrenal glands and blood sugar regulation by insulin will malfunction. Decreased intake of calories and fluid combined with progression of their underlying disease process causes weakness. When a patient significantly decreases food intake, the body conserves what nutrients it does receive and shunts the blood supply from peripheral sites to the major organs. To further conserve energy, the brain decreases the amount of time the patient

- 29 -

is awake by imposing periods of sleep. Pain medications add to fatigue and weakness. Schedule care-giving activities so the patient's energy and 'awake time' is preserved for visits by family and loved ones.

Decreased activity level

When patients are near the end of life, they experience a general slowing of body functions. Muscles lose strength and tone, and may atrophy if the patient is immobile and ROM exercises are neglected. End-stage patients often lose sensation in their extremities because of neuropathy (nerve damage). Neuropathy usually begins distally (away from the trunk) and gradually progress proximally (toward the trunk). Diabetics are especially prone to neuropathy. Patients with neuropathy will require increased assistance with mobility to avoid accidents, and more frequent position changes. The loss of muscle tone and mass places your patient at a higher risk for the development of pressure ulcers. Take care when moving your patient to prevent shearing injuries of the skin, which will be especially fragile if your patient takes steroids. Fatigue is common near the end of life. Schedule activity to minimize patient fatigue. Report changes in activity levels to the Registered Nurse.

Relaxation

The benefits of relaxation and relaxation therapy have been shown in multiple studies. The patient who actively participates in relaxation exercises is often able to significantly decrease symptoms and levels of anxiety. End-stage patients lose control over many aspects of their lives and treatment. Practicing relaxation techniques allows them to regain some control of their treatment. Relaxation has a positive effect on pain and is often able to reduce it significantly. Muscle tension, blood pressure and heart rate also respond to relaxation. Patients who are relaxed may experience an increased ability to sleep, increased effectiveness of medications, and a decrease in side effects of medication and chemotherapy. Many patients report a decrease in depression with relaxation. Some relaxation methods available are: Yoga; hypnosis; biofeedback; visualization; Feldenkrais; reflexology; and prayer. Let the patient select the best method.

Music

Classical and New Age music that is incorporated into relaxation techniques is well documented for improving emotional and physiological responses. However, every culture and subculture has its own style of music, so do not restrict your patient's listening to classical and New Age. Let your patient choose the music, even if you do not agree with his or her choice. If you dislike the music or find it too sedating, provide your patient with headphones. Keep in mind that your patient's choice may vary, depending on mood. If your patient is non-verbal, let the family and/or caregivers choose music that is comforting to the patient. Prepare your patient for relaxation prior to using music by bathing, positioning and creating a calm environment. Music the patient enjoys will decrease stress, pain, anxiety, blood pressure and heart rate. Stimulating music the patient dislikes is agitating and intensifies pain.

Recreation activities

An occupational therapist (OT) can best design a safe recreational program for your end-stage patient to distract him from anxiety and fear. Give the occupational therapist some background on your patient's cultural, gender, and religious beliefs surrounding death, so that the program is appropriate, supportive, and encouraging. Outline for the OT how and when your patient demonstrates fatigue and pain, which will limit your patient's ability to participate in activities. When the OT's plan is complete, schedule recreational activities according to your patient's needs. If an OT is unavailable, try to find a recreation leader. If you must divert your patient's attention without assistance, try journaling, reading aloud, and reviewing or creating photo albums. These activities decrease pain, lower blood pressure and heart rate, and increase the patient's sense of well-being and control. If your patient is uninterested in these activities, allow him or her to choose recreational activities and with whom to share this time.

Therapeutic massage

Many end-stage patients experience loneliness and isolation. From the moment we are born, touch is imperative for our sense of security and belonging. Friends and family, fear getting close to the debilitated patient, who is touched less and less until, for some, their only touch comes from the hands of caregivers. Therapeutic touch and massage evoke beneficial emotional and physiological responses in patients. After massage, therapy patients exhibit signs of increased circulation, decreased pain, and increased mobility. They express decreased loneliness and isolation, and the perception that they are cared for. Many patients are able to sleep soundly after a massage, which is often difficult for the Hospice and Palliative Care patient.

Therapeutic touch and energy therapy

Therapeutic Touch does not involve the physical touching of a patient's body. Therapeutic Touch is based on the belief that every person's body has fields of energy and that any alteration or interruption in the flow of one's energy causes illness. The Therapeutic Touch practitioner moves his or her hands through the energy fields of the patient in an effort to realign these fields in such a way that the patient's energy flows smoothly. This realignment promotes healing, increases relaxation, and decreases pain and anxiety. Reiki is another form of therapeutic touch that is based on the belief of energy pathways, with its origins in Buddhism. Reiki is a hands-on touch therapy, in which the practitioner realigns the flow of energy through the patient's energy fields and body to decrease pain and anxiety, and promote healing by returning the patient's energy to the proper pathways.

Compresses

Moist compresses irrigate chronic wounds to encourage healing. Dry, warm compresses relieve muscle spasms and congestion, and promote blood flow. Dry, cold compresses relieve swelling and pain by constricting blood vessels and numbing nerves. Moisture conducts heat; so moist, warm compresses have a lower temperature than dry ones. You may use commercial compresses (e.g., Aqua-K, Cara, SoftHeat, or Dunlap) or you may make salt or linseed poultices. The CNA must know the allowed procedures for compresses in the state where he or she practices.

DO	DON'T
• Check care plan to find out: Exact temperature; moist or dry application; treatment location; treatment length • Monitor application site for signs of complications: Redness (erythema); pale skin (pallor); blisters (vesicles); bluish discoloration (cyanosis) • Remove compress immediately if patient complains of numbness, burning, or pain	• Deviate from care plan • Leave hot or cold compresses in place longer than 20 minutes • Apply a compress over an area with liniment on it; to do so can cause third degree burns

Actively dying patients

Feeding
Your dying patient is not taking in adequate nutrition, so his or her metabolism changes and energy declines. When this happens, your patient will have less awake time, which can cause the family concern. Food is often associated with comfort. The family's inability to provide this comfort for their loved one can be a source of distress. The CNA can assist the family by educating them to the problems a patient may experience by consuming more than desired at this point. Your dying patient's altered metabolism means his or her body is unable to handle nutrients in a normal way. Excess food and fluid will cause an increase in respiratory and gastric secretions that can result in dyspnea, abdominal distention, pain and peripheral edema. All of these conditions put the patient at risk for infection, skin breakdown and pain.

Providing fluids
Most actively dying patients are dehydrated because they are no longer consuming adequate food and fluids, but there is little discomfort associated with this. Dehydration helps reduce nausea, vomiting, and edema for end-stage patients. The most common complaint is dry lips, nasal membranes and mouth. Oral and nasal drying often results from increased mouth breathing, medication side effects (e.g., antihistamines), and supplementary oxygen delivered by mask or nasal cannula. The family may wish to provide your patient with fluids to drink as a way to relieve suffering and offer comfort. However, the result could be to increase your patient's distress by increasing respiratory and gastrointestinal secretions. Increased secretions lead to dyspnea, abdominal pain and distention, and peripheral edema. A bloated patient is at risk for skin breakdown, infection and pain. Cleanse your patient's mouth and lips frequently with cool water or protective gel that help them retain moisture, to ease the

- 32 -

discomfort without creating more problems.

Educating the family

It is often difficult for family members to cope with the physical changes associated with the dying patient. One of the most alarming is significant weight loss and muscle wasting, called *cachexia*. Food is associated with comfort and caring. When you ask the family to withhold food, it can leave them feeling frustrated and unable to do anything to help. Reaching this point with the patient may force family members to accept that death is imminent. Educate the family about the physiological changes that take place in the dying patient to help them understand that the withholding of food is actually beneficial. The change in metabolism that results from decreased nutrition causes the body to produce and release *endorphins*, which are peptide hormones for natural pain control. Dehydration reduces the production and accumulation of secretions in the respiratory and gastrointestinal tract and reduces edema, and may decrease pain caused by the pressure tumors exert on surrounding tissues, all of which make the patient more comfortable.

Changes in bowel habits

As patients approach death, it is almost universal that their intake of food and fluids decreases. Decreased input means decreased output of urine and feces. Monitor the intake and output of patients and be aware of the signs and symptoms of constipation and urinary retention. Constipation, abdominal distention, nausea and vomiting can indicate bowel obstruction or volvulus (twisted intestine). Urinary retention can indicate kidney failure or a blockage from a stone or tumor. Diarrhea creates significant fluid loss and unbalances electrolytes; heart attack can result. Report these symptoms to the Registered Nurse immediately. Constipated patients are uncomfortable and more difficult to manage. Follow instructions in the care plan for the treatment of constipation, under the direction of the Registered Nurse.

Congestion

Patients experience increased respiratory secretions as they approach death, and are unable to clear them independently. Many experience a drowning sensation. Frequent episodes of coughing leave patients fatigued. Assist the patient with dyspnea to clear the airway by repositioning, and encourage deep breathing and coughing exercises. Use caution, because patients with osteoporosis may fracture ribs if they cough hard. Note the quality of your patient's cough – dry and non-productive, or wet and productive. If these non-invasive methods are ineffective, inform the Registered Nurse. The RN may suction the airway, and ask the doctor to prescribe antihistamines and decongestants. If the patient has a productive cough, the doctor may order you to assist the patient to collect a sputum sample. The best time is when the patient awakes, because fluid collects overnight. Wear gloves. Label the jar in ink. Open the sterile jar and ask the patient to expel lung fluid into it, *not saliva*. Cap the jar, place it in a biohazard bag, and refrigerate until pick-up by the lab.

Increased sleepiness

During the last four weeks of life, end-stage patients experience a marked increase in sleepiness due to decreased intake of calories, dehydration, hypoxia, psychological withdrawal, organ failure, and vital exhaustion. As caloric intake decreases, the body conserves energy and shunts blood flow from the periphery to the core to preserve the vital organs (brain, heart, lungs, and kidneys). Rerouting the blood supply triggers the brain to decrease the amount of time a patient is awake. Depending on the underlying disease process, the amount of awake time a patient experiences may be related to a significant decrease in oxygen availability. A low blood oxygen level (hypoxia) will result in sleepiness. For those patients receiving opiates, an increase in sleepiness occurs as a side effect of the medication. Azotemia (also called uremia) causes sleepiness as the kidneys fail. Azotemia causes death 8—12 days after a patient decides to stop dialysis. Report increased sleepiness and changes in sleep patterns to the Registered Nurse.

Agitation or restlessness

Patients experience acute agitation from urinary retention, constipation, dyspnea, medication side effects, and pain over the course of their diseases. When death is imminent in one or two days, many patients experience another final flare of agitation, which is difficult for families and caregivers to watch. It is the responsibility of the CNA to monitor the patient for signs of agitation and be prepared with appropriate interventions. The most common cause of agitation in the dying patient is pain. If your patient is non-verbal, rely on physical symptoms to determine when the patient is experiencing pain. Reposition the patient. Notify the RN that the patient needs pain medication. Divert the patient's attention

through music or reading. If the patient approaches death with fear or spiritual unrest, it may express itself as agitation. Ask if he or she wants to speak to a chaplain. Chaplains have contacts among many religions, and can arrange visits from the appropriate spiritual leader.

Signs and symptoms of end-stage disease:
- Changes in physical appearance related to the underlying disease process (e.g., cachexia, edema, and hair loss)
- Decreased function and mobility
- Significant fatigue
- Increasing periods of sleepiness
- Uncharacteristic anxiety, restlessness and fear
- Decreased consumption of food and fluids
- Increased dependency on caregivers for assistance with activities of daily living (ADL)
- Increased need for assistive devices

Loss of independence is often difficult for patients and their family. It is the responsibility of the CNA to support the patient and family through these changes by helping them understand the dying process. Generally, these signs and symptoms occur gradually, which helps patients and families to adjust.

When death is imminent

It is important that the CNA understand the cultural and religious beliefs of the patient and his or her family, because these two aspects are highlighted when death is approaching. It is the responsibility of the CNA to support the patient and family and to respect the wishes of the patient. The CNA must monitor the patient for physiological signs that indicate death is imminent, even if the patient does not complain of symptoms. Most patients within the last four weeks of life will experience significant fatigue and weakness and require additional assistance. Pain may increase in the dying patient, or the patient's requirement for pain control medication may decrease as the body releases endorphins. Endorphins are polypeptide hormones produced by the pituitary gland and hypothalamus in the brain that act as natural pain suppressants. Most patients experience difficulty breathing (dyspnea) and this is most distressing for families. Careful positioning of the patient and improving air circulation facilitates breathing.

It is the responsibility of the CNA to know the most common signs and symptoms of impending death and to provide comfort and care to the patient and family during this time. As death approaches, the most common changes in the patient are an increase in fatigue, weakness and sleepiness. These symptoms are often accompanied by a decreased need for pain medication, increased difficulty breathing (dyspnea) and marked decrease in intake of food and fluids. There may or may not be urinary and fecal incontinence. It is important that the CNA understand the cultural beliefs of the patient and family, so they can offer support through this emotional time. In some cultures, only same-sex family members are allowed to be with the dying patient when death is imminent, while others make no distinction about this. The patient's wishes are paramount and must be respected.

Use of air circulation

One of the most common symptoms at the end of life is difficulty breathing (dyspnea). While this can be related to the underlying disease process, most patients near death experience dyspnea as a result of:

- Increased respiratory secretions
- Increased breathing muscle weakness
- Decreased ability to clear respiratory secretions
- Metabolic changes that alter the effectiveness of gas exchange in the lungs

Dyspnea is often the most distressing of symptoms, as the patient fears the sensation of suffocating, and the family is concerned because they are unable to provide relief and comfort to their loved one. The easiest and least invasive way for the CNA to relieve dyspnea is to use fans to increase the circulation of air in the patient's room. Many patients report a decrease in dyspnea when they feel air moving across their faces. If fans are ineffective, inform the RN and RT that supplemental oxygen seems indicated.

Patients' belief system

Often, patients approaching death feel they have lost control of their lives, which can be as distressing as their physical symptoms. The CNA must understand the cultural, gender and religious beliefs of patients and their families. *Belief systems* play a vital role in the expectations of the patient and family members. It is also important that the CNA recognizes his or her own personal beliefs surrounding death, and does not impose his or her own belief system on the patient and family. Most patients find familiar family and/or religious objects comforting. Treat religious and family artifacts with the utmost respect. Regardless of where the patient is receiving hospice care, he or she deserves to spend time in an environment tailored to his or her preferences. A home-like environment provides comfort and security. Allow the patient to reach the end of life in peace, even if you disagree with his or her choices.

The CNA must accept how cultural and religious beliefs of the patient and family require environmental changes as death nears. You may be required to place particular objects of sentimental value or religious significance around the sick room. The schedule may change to allow for religious rites. You may be asked to assist with ritual washing and dressing. Some patients prefer quiet and few visitors. If your patient prefers to be surrounded by family and friends, you must rearrange the sick room to ensure the patient's privacy when performing personal care. Support the patient's choice of environment, whether hospice and palliative care is being given in a facility or the patient's home. Develop strategies so that your patient's choices do not interfere with those of other dying patients, such as encouraging the use of headphones. Examine your own belief systems surrounding death and do not impose your personal beliefs or preferences on the patient's environment. Respect the wishes of the patient and attempt to provide the environment the patient desires.

Nutrition and hydration
Most cultures attach significant importance to the role of consuming meals together. As patients experience the progression of disease and approach death, the goals of nutrition and hydration change. Changing feeding routines often proves distressing for patients and their families. It is the responsibility of the CNA to understand the changes and help support the patient and their family as the need for food decreases. As death approaches, the goal of eating and drinking is no longer to meet the nutritional needs of the patient. In fact, introducing food and/or fluids as the patient's organs shut down can cause or increase discomfort for the patient. End-stage patients produce increased mucous in the respiratory tract, which leads to dyspnea and the death rattle. If fluids are introduced, the body uses it to increase secretions, which causes increased respiratory difficulty. A more appropriate use of fluid is to moisten the patient's mouth for speaking.

Most cultures attach significant social importance to eating meals together and the CNA must understand the cultural background and the significance of sharing meals in that culture. As a patient approaches death, the goal of eating and drinking becomes social, rather than meeting the diminished nutritional needs of the patient. Anorexia in the patient signals that the dying process has begun. Families often exhibit distress because they perceive that the patient is starving. It is important that the CNA understands the metabolic changes occurring in the patient's body, and educates and supports the patient and family. Patients who continue to consume food after metabolic changes have started organ shutdown will experience increased edema and discomfort. End-stage patients are unable to process food comfortably, as the intestinal tract slows significantly or stops functioning altogether.

Nebulizer treatments

Nebulizer treatments are therapeutic interventions that allow the patient to inhale medication in mist form. The purpose of nebulizer treatments is to alleviate difficulty breathing (dyspnea) associated with lung diseases such as asthma, emphysema, lung cancer, and Chronic Obstructive Pulmonary Disease (COPD). Examples of nebulizer medication are Pulmicort Respules (budesonide) and Atrovent (ipratropium). Some states do not permit CNAs to administer medication. It is the responsibility of every CNA to know the regulations regarding medication administration in the state in which they practice. The CNA can assist the Registered Nurse in nebulizer administration by preparing the patient for treatment. This includes positioning the patient, cleaning and assembling the nebulizer apparatus, and encouraging the patient in deep breathing and coughing exercises prior to and after treatment. The CNA must recognize side effects of nebulizer therapy, like slow clinical response that can require a switch to IV.

Inhalers

Inhalers are devices that allow the patient to inhale medication directly into the lungs. Direct administration provides for rapid absorption and action of the medication. Examples of inhaled medications are Flovent (fluticasone propionate) and Ventolin (salbutamol). It is the responsibility of the CNA to know the regulations for medication administration in the state of practice. Regardless of the state in which the CNA practices, the CNA may assist the Registered Nurse in the administration of inhaled medications by:

- Keeping the inhaler apparatus accessible
- Cleaning and assembling accessory equipment, like Trudelle's AeroChamber
- Preparing the patient with breathing exercises
- Positioning the patient appropriately
- Explaining the procedure to the patient, so he or she is ready to use the inhaler
- Monitoring the patient for side-effects of the medication the patient receives through the inhaler

PD&P

Postural drainage and chest percussion (PD&P) is an airway clearance technique to alleviate dyspnea. PD&P helps the patient move mucus out of the lungs and into the upper respiratory tract, where it can be coughed out. Patients with restricted breathing from recurrent lung infection or excess mucous have *bronchiectasis.* Diseases that cause bronchiectasis and require PD&P include: Cystic fibrosis; infections with *Bordetella pertussis, Klebsiella,* or *Staphylococcus*; Young's syndrome; and Kartagener's syndrome. The caregiver repeatedly and rhythmically taps the patient's chest and back with cupped hands. Correctly performed chest percussion produces a characteristic hollow sound. If a slapping sound is heard, the procedure is being performed incorrectly. If the patient cannot cough up mucous independently, the RN suctions it to clear the airway and allow air to flow into and out of the lungs. Trained family members may perform

PD&P. Some patients prefer to have the CNA perform PD&P. The CNA must know the state laws pertaining to therapeutic interventions like PD&P where he or she practices.

Grief

Grief is a normal response to the death of a loved one. How a person deals with grief is very personal, and each person will grieve differently. Elisabeth Kubler-Ross identified these five stages of grief in her book *On Death and Dying*:
- Denial — This can't be happening
- Anger — Why me!
- Bargaining — I'll do anything if...
- Depression — I just can't handle it
- Acceptance — Everything will be all right

A person may not necessarily follow the stages in order, or go through each stage. A person should go through at least two of the five stages. Patients who have been battling a disease may be willing to accept death to avoid pain, but may not be ready to leave their family and friends for the unknown of death. Family members may disagree on the patient's choice to allow death to occur. Expect conflict and tension as they struggle with loss. Support the patient and family but do not impose your personal ideals or beliefs for end-of-life care.

Psychosocial and Spiritual Care

Spiritual needs

Complex emotions are evoked by death and dying, and many of these emotions have their basis in spirituality. Your patient they may find comfort or discomfort in spirituality, depending on his or her cultural and religious beliefs and background. Patients who follow a spiritual belief that assures peace and reunion with loved ones after death often face their demise with less anxiety than those who believe in punishment for sins or no afterlife (e.g., atheists and humanists). Your patient may want to make atonement or do penance for sins. Your patient may refuse treatment because of his or her spiritual beliefs (e.g., Jehovah's Witnesses and Christian Scientists). It is the responsibility of the CNA to understand the culture and spiritual beliefs of the patient and family. Most patients and families are very willing to share this information with the caregivers. It brings them comfort to know the patient's wishes will be understood and respected. Regardless of the CNA's personal beliefs, the patient's wishes and beliefs must be respected.

Identifying spiritual issues

End-of-life care is an emotional and stressful time for patients and their families, who often confide their feelings to the CNA. A primary motive for divulging personal feelings to an outsider is to avoid distressing the patient and other family members. When the patient and family bring their fears, cares, and concerns to your attention, view them in the context of their cultural and spiritual background. The CNA functions within the intimate space of the patient. Often, no other confidante is present. It is important that the CNA has sufficient knowledge to offer comfort at the end of life. Determine with the patient which areas of concern may be shared with others, and which should remain in confidence. The CNA is responsible for knowing the state law regarding mandatory reporting of abuse and neglect.

Guilt

A common pattern seen in dying patients is for them to spend time reviewing their lives. As they reminisce, patients commonly report feelings of guilt associated with actions performed or omitted, or over relationships that were less than ideal. Patients often report guilt for leaving their families with financial burdens related to medical care. A patient may feel guilty about leaving the family with tasks for which the patient feels responsible. It is often the CNA who hears of these feelings, not the persons directly involved. Consider the information revealed to you in the family's cultural and spiritual context. Be aware of sources of guidance both for yourself and the patient, such as Chaplaincy and Social Work. Connect the patient and family with resources to help them manage strong emotions. Doctors, nurses, pharmacists, and social workers are legally bound to report some offenses, such as child and elder neglect or abuse, rape, and murder. You must know if your state's law makes you a mandatory reporter, also.

Chaplain support

Chaplaincy can arrange for spiritual visitors in your patient's religion of choice, and can provide standard religious texts, like the Bible, Koran, Book of Mormon, and Talmud. Chaplains are trained in psychology, multiculturalism, ethics, disaster management, and pandemic issues. They have strong ties to Social Work, and can find community resources quickly. If the CNA requires cultural and spiritual background to treat the patient and family correctly, then a chaplain is an excellent resource to tap. The CNA is not required to share or agree with the belief system of the patient and family, just to respect it at all times and schedule care to facilitate religious practices. Many patients and their families will discuss personal spiritual issues related to death and dying with the CNA. If they present information that they wish to remain strictly confidential (e.g., a confession), the CNA must know how to reach the chaplain on-call for support.

Permission to die

Some dying patients require permission to die. Your patient may struggle to remain alive due to fear of the unknown or spiritual unrest. Your patient may feel his or her life's work is incomplete. Your patient may cling to life because of the hardship his or her death will cause the family, such as a patient who will leave behind young children who require care. If your patient falls into one of these categories, give them permission to let go and allow death to occur. This may be a task that is too difficult for a family member and if so, the CNA may be called upon to speak to the patient about it. If you are uncomfortable doing this, most Hospice and Palliative Care programs offer training in this area. If you need help with sensitive phrasing, contact a chaplain or psychologist.

Respecting differences

The CNA becomes involved in intimate dynamics when providing care for the Hospice and Palliative Care patient and grieving family. As a healthcare professional with privileged access, the

CNA must perform his or her duties confidentially, and provide excellent care without judgment or disrespect. Respect extends to gender issues, politics, lifestyle choices, and religious doctrine. Your patient may suffer from a stigmatized disease, like AIDS or syphilis. The CNA must advocate for the patient. It is not necessary for the CNA to agree with the patient and family, but it is necessary that the CNA respect their wishes regarding the care of the patient and rituals for the approach of death. The family may be embroiled in a legal battle over the death, e.g., Jehovah's Witnesses refuse blood transfusions. Recognize that your patient's cultural and spiritual background and attitudes affect the care plan and medical approach. Most Hospice and Palliative Care programs provide diversity training.

Multicultural issues

Check your policies & procedures manual for instructions about how to deal with multicultural issues. If the manual does not cover the specific issue you need, contact a chaplain for advice. The CNA needs to know the patient's cultural and religious background to provide excellent care, even if the patient is non-verbal. Most Hospice and Palliative Care programs provide multicultural or sensitivity training. Most patients and their families are willing to share their beliefs, so do not be embarrassed to ask about their preferences. The peri-death period increases anxiety and stress. When the patient and family follow familiar cultural and religious rituals and practices, it makes death into a rite of passage and decreases stress significantly. Allow the family as much latitude as possible, without causing undue stress for your other patients. If

you anticipate that a ritual will be noisy or alarming for other patients, respectfully guide the family to the Quiet Room. Move other patients out of the area for ritual washing and vigils.

Death and dying are emotionally charged events. Your patient's family members may disagree with the care plan, or the doctor's decision not to tube feed or resuscitate the patient (DNR). *All* members of the interdisciplinary team should facilitate effective communication and offer resources. However, since the CNA spends the most time with the patient and family, it frequently falls to the CNA. Understand how the patient's cultural and spiritual background impacts family dynamics, for example:

- In patriarchal Mexican culture, the eldest male speaks for the patient
- Muslim females resist care by males
- Asian Americans and American Indians are reserved and dislike highly personal questions
- Western Europeans are action-oriented and more likely to want interventions
- Fatalistic cultures disapprove of interventions
- Cultures with a circular time perspective are unconcerned with schedules

Use *appropriate* humor to help people deal with absurd events and bizarre behavior in a healthy manner. Therapeutic humor reinforces the family's learning and enhances their performance when you teach them patient care.

Religious and spiritual customs

Your patient may be too ill to attend regular religious services. Tune in the TV or radio to broadcast services of your patient's choice. Arrange for the chaplain to hold a bedside service, or bring your patient to the chapel for a non-denominational service. Discuss with the patient and family their particular customs surrounding death and dying, particularly if the patient is in an in-patient facility. If they want to enact traditional ceremonies, relay this information to the proper authorities at your facility well before death takes place. Advocate for allowing the patient's wishes to be honored. Many ceremonies involve the use of candles or incense. All patient care facilities have strict fire regulations. Smoke may irritate other patients' lungs. If your facility cannot accommodate the patient's traditions, make the patient, family, and chaplain or religious visitor aware as early as possible, to avoid conflict later.

Death brings with it multiple emotional and spiritual stressors, so it is important that the patient and family are allowed to follow their cultural and spiritual beliefs associated with death. The patient and family are most likely to turn to the CNA to discuss their concerns, because the CNA is the most visible member of the healthcare team, who functions in the intimate space of the patient and family. Other caregivers are more remote and may seem less approachable. Many cultures and religions share a belief in the transition to an afterlife. Often, there are specific practices that must take place to assure the patient's place in the next life. If the medical staff does not follow the family's spiritual beliefs, it increases anxiety and stress for both the patient and family. The CNA helps reduce stress by advocating for the spiritual needs of the patient and family.

Patient relationships

The CNA must show respect for the relationships patients have with their families and friends. You may not approve of dominance, financial, or gender roles that surface, but it is unnecessary for you to agree. If your patient's situation conflicts with your own personal belief system and you cannot act respectfully in good conscience, then you must ask your supervisor to remove you from the case, and wait until you are relieved of duty. If you suspect abuse or neglect, notify the Registered Nurse. If state law makes you a mandatory reporter, check your policies & procedure manual to find out the correct reporting procedure. All Hospice and Palliative Care programs offer training on how to handle these reportable offenses: Assault; arson; killing by accident, assisted suicide, self-defense, insanity or murder; bomb or death threats; kidnapping, confining, and restraining; possession of a controlled substance in violation of law; possession of an illegal weapon or explosive; sexual offenses; robbery; abuse; and neglect.

Socio-economic background

The Hospice and Palliative Care movement holds that every patient has the right to die with dignity and be cared for throughout the dying process with respect. This belief extends not only to the patient, but also to the grieving family. It is important that the CNA understands the socioeconomic background of the patient, because it limits or extends the resources available to assist the patient and family through the dying process. It is inadvisable for a CNA to witness a will, because he or she can be accused of exerting undue influence over the patient, or the end-stage patient's mental status may be questioned. Financial background also pertains to the cultural and spiritual belief system of the patient and family. Some cultures place significant spiritual importance on wealth and its meaning in the afterlife. Regardless of where the patient and family are in the spectrum of socioeconomics, it is the responsibility of the CNA to treat all patients and their families equally, with respect and dignity, and without prejudice.

Treatment choices

Regardless of the CNA's personal opinion, it is his or her responsibility as a healthcare professional and member of the interdisciplinary Hospice and Palliative Care Team to support and respect the choices made by the patient and family. If the family's choices conflict with the CNA's strong personal opinions related to end-of-life care, then the CNA must terminate care, after giving *adequate written notice* to the patient and physician to avoid charges of patient abandonment. The CNA is legally required to wait until relieved by another member of the healthcare team who has equal or greater training. Examples of common conflicts that arise are:

- Tube feeding to prolong life when a patient can no longer eat independently
- Parents refuse blood transfusions, pain relief, and treatments for minors
- Safety hazards (e.g., a dangerous dog, sexual harassment, or threats)
- Patient will not or cannot pay bills because of insurance problems
- Patient is unruly and obnoxious

Identifying support needs

The CNA is with the patient and family for extended periods of time. Patients and families become familiar with and relaxed around the CNA. The CNA is in a unique position to observe behaviors over time. Here are common examples of behaviors that should alert the CNA to a need for added support:

Behavior	Solution
The patient asks questions about what happens after death	The CNA arranges a visit by a chaplain
Family members show concern about the financial burden of burial costs and childcare	The CNA contacts a Social Worker
The patient expresses boredom, and has increased signs of pain	The CNA arranges for the public library's bookmobile to deliver books, videos, and music

The CNA should discuss any issues of concern with the Registered Nurse.

Resources and education

Approach of death
The CNA is the member of the healthcare team who spends the greatest amount of time with the patient and family, so it often falls to the CNA to have conversations with them regarding death. Remember that the family's cultural and spiritual background have significant impact on how they process information about death. Answer all questions from the patient and family openly and honestly. If you do not know the correct answer, discuss the issue with the appropriate member of the healthcare team and be certain to get answers in a

timely manner. If you are uncomfortable with any discussions, relay their concerns to the Registered Nurse. Hospice and Palliative Care programs offer training and resources for staff, families and patients regarding issues related to death. Keep a current list of contact numbers ready to help your patients.

Agency services and community resources

Be aware of the many national and local resources available for Hospice and Palliative Care patients and their families. Visit the National Hospice and Palliative Care Organization (NHPCO) at http://www.nhpco.org for information on diseases, organ donation, Medicare rights, the U.S. Living Will Registry, and caring for children and the aged. Local services and resources vary widely; find out who is responsible for maintaining up-to-date information at your hospice. It is not your responsibility to know all the programs available, because research reduces your time for patient care. However, you are responsible for relaying the needs of the patient and family to the appropriate person, to ensure they have access to all resources. If you are aware of an unmet need, but do not know the appropriate person, relay concerns to the Registered Nurse. Explain the cultural and spiritual background of the patient to the resource person. Present information from the resource person to the family in context with their beliefs, to make them more receptive to help.

Grief and loss counseling

The CNA often spends more time with the Hospice and Palliative Care patient and family than any other member of the healthcare team, and is in a position to educate the family about grief and loss, or arrange for counseling. Answer questions regarding grief and loss openly, honestly, and in the cultural and spiritual context of the patient. Ensure the source of the information you give the family is reputable. Do not give your patients written material that is more than five years old because it is probably obsolete. The National Hospice and Palliative Care Organization (NHPCO) is a reliable resource for correct and up-to-date information. Direct the patient's and family's questions to the appropriate internal resource if you are unable to answer their questions (e.g., chaplain, psychologist, social worker, RN, attending physician, or librarian). Arrange for a translator, if needed. Be clear about your own emotions surrounding death, because it will color your response to the patient.

Energy-saving techniques

End-stage patients experience significant fatigue, which increases as death approaches. Metabolic changes, disease progression, decreased nutrient and fluid intakes, and aging contribute to fatigue. Consider the impact physical exertion has on the dying patient and schedule activities accordingly. An exhausted caregiver is unable to provide good care. Educate the family caregivers regarding techniques that allow them and the patient to conserve energy:

- Perform personal care at the most active time, often the morning
- Work in an efficient manner, with all equipment within reach to prevent delays or interruptions in care
- Combine tasks to save energy for visiting time
- Arrange respite care and take regular breaks

- Use assistive devices, and ensure they have the right settings

Nutrition and hydration

Most end-stage patients decrease the amount of food and fluid they consume spontaneously, to avoid nausea and decrease edema and mucous. Hunger and dehydration are uncomfortable for a healthy person, but actually benefit the dying patient. Decreased nutrition causes metabolic changes, meaning the patient has less 'awake time' and an increased release of endorphins, the body's natural painkillers (analgesics). The CNA must understand these principles and explain them to the family so they are aware of and accept changes taking place in their loved one. Your patient's family may resist a care plan with calorie and fluid restrictions because of their cultural background. Ask the RN to have the attending physician speak with them about it.

Personal care and comfort measures

Your patient must consent to allowing family members to provide personal care. Many family members want to participate in the physical care of the dying patient, but require training in how to provide excellent care. The CNA teaches family caregivers to avoid falls, aspiration, and skin tears by rehearsing safe lifting and positioning techniques with them. The CNA must demonstrate proper body mechanics for the caregiver, and a variety of positions for the patient to relieve specific problems. For example, patients with ascites benefit from Sim's position, and patients with dyspnea benefit from Fowler's position. Emphasize skin care, positioning and turning the patient, and timing care in association with pain medication and periods of fatigue. Know the limits of practice allowed in your state. Refer the family to the Registered Nurse for instruction on activities out of the scope of the CNA practice.

Reframing hope

Dying patients and their family members experience loss of hope when they realize death is unavoidable. Significant emotion is involved in making the decision to accept Hospice and Palliative Care. Patients and families struggle with the meaning of palliative care. They may not absorb a verbal explanation when they are initially upset. The World Health Organization (WHO) provides an excellent definition of palliative care at: http://www.who.int/cancer/palliative/definition/en/print.html. It is multiculturally sensitive and inoffensive to people of most spiritual backgrounds. Offer a print copy to the patient and family to explain palliative care. Allow the dying patient and grieving family to work through feelings of hopelessness. Focus on the patient's positive achievements. In palliative care, the hope is not that the patient will be cured, but that the patient's pain is well managed to enhance quality of life. It may be difficult for some patients and their families to shift their focus. Consistently demonstrate by example that hope remains.

Isolation protocols

Follow the isolation protocol that the Infection Control Practitioner posts on your patient's door *exactly*. This means hand washing before and after patient contact, donning *all* the personal protective equipment (PPE) listed on the door *every time*, and disposing of garbage in biohazard containers for incineration. Your employer is obligated by law to ensure you receive extensive training regarding medical isolation protocols, and to provide free PPE. Isolation protocols are unfamiliar and frightening for the patient and visitors. Educate the patient and visitors about isolation, and ensure that they follow correct technique to avoid spreading communicable diseases. Isolation protocols vary, based on either the patient's infection or the patient's susceptibility to contracting an infection (reverse isolation for immunosuppressed patients). Although isolation is distressing for the patient and family because it separates them from their normal contact, you must enforce it consistently as a job requirement.

Respite care

Some palliative care patients have direct personal care provided by family members or close friends, assisted by the healthcare team. Homecare may prove exhausting for the family. Their own illness, injury, or life events may interfere with their ability to provide care. When this happens, the patient needs respite care. The doctor may dispatch a CNA, RN, and physiotherapist to the home, and order supplies delivered from a local pharmacy. The care team will arrange meal and cleaning services. If the patient deteriorates, the doctor may decide to admit the patient to a hospice, nursing home, or hospital. The family may view these changes as personal failures, and may feel they have let the patient down. The CNA and healthcare team must provide excellent patient care, and support and educate the family caregivers in the context of their cultural background.

Patient rights

A patient advocate speaks on the patient's behalf to obtain services and information, and protect rights. If your institution works on the case management system, it will appoint an advocate for each patient, usually an RN or Social Worker. The CNA spends more time with the dying patient than the case manager. Relate the hopes, wishes, fears and concerns of the patient to the healthcare team. Do not become embroiled in emotional family dynamics by revealing confidences. However, expressing the patient's desires through the healthcare team is an appropriate avenue to ensure the patient's voice is heard. The American Hospital Association replaced its *Patients' Bill of Rights* in April 2008 with a brochure called *The Patient Care Partnership*, available in many languages. Obtain a free copy for your patient at http://www.aha.org.

Communication barriers

The CNA is the team member who spends the most time with the patient and family, and is in the best position to observe communication problems. Once the CNA identifies a problem, he or she is responsible for relaying information to the interdisciplinary team and seeking resources to enhance communication. For example, the CNA may:
- Recommend that the family receives interpreter services
- Report that the patient is withdrawn, fearful, and silent in the presence of certain family members

Communication barriers include:
- *Inappropriate Language:* Criticism; name-calling; ordering; moralizing; threatening; excessive

questioning; minimizing problems; diagnosing & offering unqualified advice

- *Physical Barriers:* Tracheostomy tubes; background noise; deafness; ill-fitting face masks; patient response changed by drugs; speech impediment; psychiatric disorders
- *System Design Flaws:* Inadequate staffing; staff do not read chart or take report at beginning of shift; lack of multicultural sensitivity training; no interpreters
- *Attitudinal Barriers:* Disgust; lack of motivation; personality conflict; refusal to communicate; resistance to change

As the patient progresses toward death, his or her needs change. The care plan is revised by the interdisciplinary healthcare team to meet the changing needs. The CNA is responsible for reading all updates to the care plan, and explaining the changes to the patient and family. The changes in the care plan may relate to any aspect of care, such as pain management, incontinence, or using different mattresses to reduce pressure ulcers. Initially, the goal of pain management may be to keep the patient reasonably comfortable, but awake enough to interact with family and friends. As death approaches and pain increases, the plan may change to improve comfort and increase sedation. The initial goal for patients receiving chemotherapy is to eliminate cancer. Once the patient is in Palliative Care, the goal of chemotherapy changes to slowing the growth of tumors, rather than eliminate them.

CNA as link
The CNA is the link that connects the interdisciplinary Hospice and Palliative Care Team with the patient, mediating and advocating in the patient's best interest. The patient and family often feel more relaxed with the CNA than the other team members, because they spend more time together. The family tends to ask questions related to death and dying of the CNA. The CNA is responsible for providing answers to the patient and family. If the CNA is unable to answer their questions, he or she must access resources and consult the interdisciplinary team to obtain answers. Tell the patient that you do not know, but will find out, and return with the answer in a reasonable amount of time. Questions and concerns related to death and dying are time-sensitive, emotionally charged, and may be difficult for the patient and family to ask. Frame your answer in vocabulary the patient and family will understand, and that does not offend their cultural and religious background.

Initiating conversations
Facilitate conversation among your clients who are reluctant to broach an issue, when a problem will result if they ignore it. Examples of pressing issues are pain control, childcare, and funeral expenses. Remember, your clients perceive you as safe and approachable, in contrast to more remote members of the interdisciplinary team.

- Make a personal introduction to 'break the ice' and use your first name
- Compliment those involved to make them feel positive about you (e.g., "I can see you take very good care of your grandmother, because

she has no bedsores and is always clean when I get here."
- Ask open questions that require more than a 'yes' or 'no' answer
- Offer a brochure about the thorny issue and respectfully request that they consider the information
- Offer to book an appointment with the Social Worker, who is trained in facilitating difficult discussions

Print free PEACE brochures about sensitive end-of-life issues from the American College of Physicians at http://www.acponline.org.

Body image changes

Dying patients undergo significant physical changes as death approaches. Changes result from disease process or from disfiguring treatments, like:
- Amputation
- Chemotherapy that causes hair loss
- Radiation therapy that causes burns or tattoo marks that indicate the radiation area
- Massive weight loss and muscle wasting (cachexia)

All these physical expressions of disease are distressing for your patient. The CNA is welcomed into the patient's intimate space and should support the patient as his or her body image changes. Acknowledge the patient's distress and do not minimize his or her concerns. Get a video from Look Good Feel Better (LGFB) at 1-800-395-LOOK or http://www.lookgoodfeelbetter.org to learn how to disguise the worst effects. Refer the patient to a trained counselor.

Massive weight loss and muscle wasting is called *cachexia*. It is not the same as starvation. Starving patients slow down their use of nutrients, but patients with cachexia have an increased need for vitamins, protein, and calories to fight disease. Cachexia can result from a disease process, like diabetes or AIDS, or can result from dehydration (water loss) and anorexia (lack of appetite). Cachexia changes the patient's body image and distresses the family. Many African and Indian cultures equate fat with success, health, wealth, and respect. Thin people are considered mean, sickly, neglected, and poor. Explain to the family that the dehydrated patient has less painful edema, and that restricting the diet to small, bland meals makes digestion easier. Heavy, spicy food nauseates dying patients. Weight loss is confirmation that death is approaching. Pay careful attention to skin care to prevent skin ulcers and tears as the subcutaneous fat is lost. Arrange for a dietician to assess the patient's diet and suggest changes.

Disfiguring surgical procedures
Your dying patient may undergo a disfiguring surgical procedures intended to prolong life. Surgical procedures that radically change body image include:
- Mastectomy (breast removal)
- Limb or facial amputations
- Ostomy (creation of an abdominal opening that drains urine or feces into a plastic bag)

Many other surgeries significantly change a patient's internal body, but these three external surgeries distress patients and their families the most. The family may not be able to afford a prosthesis or reconstructive surgery to make the disfigurement less visible. The patient may be too weak to relearn walking, or the skin may be too damaged to tolerate prosthesis. Both may be disgusted by the smell and mess of an ostomy. Support the patient and family as they adjust to these changes by:

- Acknowledging their feelings about the changes
- Encouraging them to express themselves
- Contacting the appropriate agency for information and funding applications

Meaning and purpose

End-stage patients and their families explore philosophical questions regarding the meaning of life as death approaches. Families faced with the loss of a loved one need to find value in their loved one's life and share that value with others. The dying patient commonly spends time trying to determine if life had a meaning and purpose, and that he or she fulfilled that purpose. It is important that the CNA understands the cultural and spiritual background of the patient and family, as the answers to these questions are based in their belief system. It is not necessary that the CNA agree with the patient and family's belief system, but their wishes must be respected at all times. Refer the patient and family to resources specialists, such as Chaplaincy, Psychiatry, Social Work, and Foundation.

If your end-stage patient is conscious, coherent, and an adult, he or she will review life and search for meaning. Often, the patient's family seeks purpose and meaning, too. Create opportunities for the patient and family work together on their search for meaning. Remember that the patient's cultural and spiritual background affects the way he or she perceives meaning. Some cultures see passing along a wealthy inheritance as proof of a good life. Others see relinquishing the desire for wealth as a spiritual triumph. Your patient may desire to give donations, make a pilgrimage, or make a confession and do penance. Access your hospice's resources to help the patient and family through this process. Observe the patient and family for indications they are ready for this activity. If they begin too early, the patient and family will not be ready to avail themselves of opportunities, and your suggestions may cause added stress and anxiety.

Visual life review projects
When your patient is ready for a life review, suggest he or she begins by looking at old photos and home movies. These are often a source of happiness and encourage recitation of memories and favorite times during family life. Most people are apt to take photographs of happy times. Provide a photo album or scrapbook for the patient and family to put together. The album offers an opportunity for the patient to relive fond memories with the family, and he or she can review it independently when they are unavailable. Remember that very young children think death is reversible, and you may have to remind them again and again that someone in the pictures is not coming back. Emphasize that the person who died did not go away because he was angry with the child, and that the doctors could not prevent the death. Assure the child that someone will take care of him when your patient dies.

Journaling or telling a life story

The end-stage patient and family need to review their life together to identify its meaning. Obtain a journal and writing materials for your patient. If your patient wants newspaper clippings to include in the journal, contact a librarian about how to obtain them. Your patient may initially be hesitant to review his or her life with others, but as he begins to trust you, will probably do so willingly. Ask the family for their assistance, because they shared many of the events with the patient, and may have supplemental information. Use your hospice's program resources and guides to assist the patient and family capture their memories. If the patient is too weak to write, borrow a tape recorder or get a volunteer to take dictation. The patient may want to preserve favorite memories as a gift for family members, or write explanations, and this is therapeutic for all concerned.

Creating an audio or video legacy

End-stage patients want to ascribe meaning to their lives. Life review happens in most cultures. Ask a librarian to inspire your patient with an autobiography from an author with the same cultural and spiritual background. If your patient wishes to leave an audio legacy, obtain the resources from your recreation director or occupational therapist. Schedule recording for a time when the patient has the most energy and will be able to participate fully. If the patient desires to create a video for family or friends, make certain the patient is groomed appropriately. Find out how to disguise illness with makeup through Look Good Feel Better, which donates complimentary tool kits and teaches patients how to use hair alternatives, prosthetic clothing, and cosmetics. Help your patient call family members or friends to arrange a film debut. If they cannot attend in person, ask your IT manager how to broadcast the movie over an Internet connection.

Phone calls and internet chats

End-stage patients may miss family and friends who do not live locally, or are unable to be physically present. Facilitate communication between the patient and family members or friends because saying a final 'good-bye' is psychologically important for closure. Use technology to your patient's advantage. Your patient may be unable to afford long distance calls over a conventional phone. If your patient does not have an e-mail account, get one free through Hotmail or Yahoo. Ask your recreation director, occupational therapist, or librarian to show the patient how to use e-mail, chat, and VOIP to make free or low-cost long distance calls over the Internet. The Internet requires little energy expenditure from the patient, and instantaneous communication brings much comfort. Arrange time on your facility's computers to correspond to the time when your patient has the most energy, even if that means interrupting the usual schedule for the day. Your patient may make new friends on-line with similar illnesses.

Safety

The interdisciplinary healthcare team must be aware of anything that threatens a dying patient's safety, whether blatant or subtle. Gangs often plant members as hospital workers to relay a patient's location, if he is likely to testify against them. Find out if your state's laws make you a mandatory reporter of abuse and neglect. If you are not a mandatory reporter, but suspect wrongdoing, report to the doctor, RN, pharmacist, or social worker. If you suspect any patient or family member is in immediate danger, call Security and 911. Patient safety is the responsibility of every healthcare professional. Harm can be: Written or verbal threats; physical attacks; tampering with medication or equipment; coercion; theft; or emotional harm. Be cautious and avoid becoming embroiled in family dynamics, but err on the side of caution and protect your patient at all times. If the threat comes from one of your colleagues, report it immediately to Human Resources, the Nurse Manager, Security Manager, or Counsel, as appropriate.

Reporting abuse

Most states require all members of the healthcare profession to report suspicions of patient abuse. If you are not satisfied that your supervisor who received the report relayed your suspicion to the proper authorities, then file a report independently. Physical, sexual, and emotional abuse may be perpetrated by the patient's family, a friend, or a healthcare professional. Look for these common signs of abuse:

- Unexplained injuries or bruises
- Sudden changes in the Will or finances
- The patient acts afraid of a particular person or situation
- The abuser gives the patient threatening looks, and limits access to the phone and finances
- The abuser yells or uses degrading language to make the patient feel guilty
- Prescriptions are unfilled or given incorrectly

The District of Columbia, American Samoa, Northern Mariana Islands, and 14 other states allow reasonable physical discipline of a child if it does not cause bodily injury.

Neglect

Neglect is habitual lack of proper food, shelter, clothing, supervision, and medical care. In some states, neglect is also: Manufacturing, storing, or using a controlled substance around a child; taking a controlled substance that impairs your ability to attend to someone in your care; and giving a child or fetus alcohol or illegal drugs. The District of Columbia and 11 states do *not* consider financial inability to care for a dependent as neglect. Caregivers who fail to leave their names and contact information are neglectful. Monitor these signs of neglect and report it:

- Dirty, ragged clothing, or dressing inappropriately for the weather
- Unattended patient
- Constant hunger, stealing food, searching trash for food, or bolting food when in a group
- Untreated medical conditions
- Dehydration and fluids are not within reach
- Incorrect positioning (bedsores, dyspnea)
- Patient is not allowed to use the bathroom
- Patient is dirty and unbathed
- Patient is isolated in a room, or not allowed visitors, phone calls, or Internet use

Substance abuse

One in 10 people have a substance abuse problem. Your dying patient may live with a substance abuser and they may be strongly attached. The substance abuser may be another member of the healthcare team, or the patient. The CNA must report substance abuse, as the dying patient's safety is threatened if an addict, alcoholic, or drug seller has access to the patient's medications or finances. Stay alert for these signs of substance abuse:

- Narcotics and syringes disappear from the sick room (OxyContin, morphine, fentanyl)
- Poor work performance, memory, concentration, or judgment
- Watery, glassy eyes; dilated or pin-point pupils
- Changes in personal grooming, appetite, and weight
- Clumsiness; slurred speech; difficulty walking; impaired vision
- Loud voice and inappropriate laughter or withdrawn and sleepy at odd times
- Mood swings and personality changes (agitated, aggressive, irritable, paranoid, unmotivated)
- Many solvent spray cans, bottles, or drug paraphernalia in the trash
- Needle tracks, drug smells, sniffling, coughing, sweating, and vomiting

Caregiver burnout

Family members often want to participate in the care of dying patients. However, if they are untrained, frail, elderly, poor, or have other pressing obligations, this participation proves overwhelming. Remember, the family is already suffering emotional distress and spiritual unrest from anticipating the death of their loved one. Observe the family for these indicators of burnout and inability to provide quality care:

- Bedsores on the patient
- Complaints of exhaustion, illness, or injury from the caregivers

- Errors in patient care (e.g., wrong medication given at the wrong time or by the wrong method)
- Irritability toward the patient and blaming the patient for the situation
- Refusal to leave when the CNA arrives to provide relief

The CNA spends much time with the patient and family, and is in a position to determine when the family needs further assistance. Explain to the family that burnout is to be expected, and inability to provide complex care is not a failure.

Final hours of life

The CNA is an important member of the healthcare team throughout the process leading to death, and often develops significant bonds with the patient and family. Many patients and families prefer the presence of a CNA in the final hours of a patient's life, rather than a doctor or nurse, because of the close, consistent care-giving relationship. Some patients and families prefer to share those last moments privately. Accept whatever the patient and family choose. The presence of the CNA can be beneficial, as it provides the patient and family with immediate access to a member of the healthcare team who can answer questions regarding the actual process of death. The CNA ensures everybody has a seat, points out where washroom, telephone, and cafeteria facilities are located, and offers to remain with the patient when family members need a break. If asked to be present, the CNA intervenes only as necessary, out of respect for the family's need for time with their loved one.

The interdisciplinary healthcare team prepares patients and their families for the imminent death of the patient. Nevertheless, the actual event is a time of great emotion. *If specific rituals cannot be conducted in your facility because they are against regulations, ensure the family understands the limitations prior to the death.* Ensure that the patient and family are treated with dignity and respect prior to and after death occurs. Check the patient's vital signs. Record the time vital signs are absent in the patient's chart. Notify the RN. If death occurred in a hospice, the nurse pronounces death. If death occurred at home, the CNA notifies the doctor, who comes to legally pronounce death and complete the death certificate. Do not begin post mortem care until after death is officially pronounced. Offer family caregivers the opportunity to assist in preparing the body if their cultural and religious traditions require participation in post mortem care. The body must be prepared before 2 hours elapse, when decomposition and rigor mortis start.

The CNA must recognize these signs of imminent death and educate the family:
- Unexpected energy and alertness a day or two before death
- Glassy eyes with dilated pupils
- Cyanosis (blue-gray skin) on the lips, hands and feet
- Cold hands and feet
- Open mouth with Cheyne-Stokes or death rattle breathing
- Unresponsiveness to voice or pain

If it appears death will occur while you are present, alert the family. Assist with contacting family members who are not present, and gathering those that are together. If visitors are tiring the patient, notify the nurse. Close the curtain around the patient for privacy. Your patient is your top priority. Encourage family members to enter behind the curtain and speak to the patient singly or in pairs, if this is allowed under the family's customs and they wish to be present. Respect the family's specific religious or cultural observances surrounding the moment of death. If family members choose to remain outside the room, relay information to them as necessary.

After death

Preparing body after death

Equipment	Procedure
Shroud kit	Close door or draw curtain
Gloves	Close patient's eyes or cover with moist gauze
Gown	Cap or clamp lines & deflate catheters
Face shield	Bathe body
Paper tape	Tape lines & catheters to body
4X4 gauze	Change bed sheets
Underpads	Pad buttocks & draining areas
Bath items	Raise head of bed 30° to reduce livor
Syringe for	Place body in supine position & straighten limbs
deflating balloon	Insert dentures & apply chin strap
catheter	Apply clean gown & toe tag
Clamps	Comb hair
Scissors	List, bag, & tag personal effects & give to family or Cashier
	Apply & tag shroud after family leaves
	Get body to Morgue for refrigeration within 2 hours, or bring to Autopsy

Regulations regarding rituals

Observe the family's cultural and religious practices to the extent possible and allow them to help with post mortem care if they want, and it was the wish of the patient. Americans and Africans clean and groom the body for a spiritual journey. The family may be forbidden to mention the patient by name. If the family's particular customs contravene the regulations of your facility, explain this to family *prior* to death to avoid a confrontation when emotions run high after death. Your institution probably will not permit things like self-mutilation, cutting of the corpse, sexual images, or ritual food placed on the corpse in any circumstances. However, many facilities will make minor exceptions regarding death rituals if the family asks the Nurse Manager for permission *beforehand*. Chanting, smoke, or processions will disturb other patients, so ask the Nurse Manager for a secluded place to move the body.

Bereavement resources

The *entire* interdisciplinary team is responsible for providing the patient's family with access to bereavement resources.

However, the family is mostly likely to ask the CNA for this information. Obtain information about bereavement resources in your community from:

- Your Hospice and Palliative Care instructor
- Bereavement group leaders within your facility
- Information packets for bereaved families prepared by your facility's educators
- Counselors' contact numbers posted in the nursing station

If your patient's family members do not live locally, direct them to national contact information through the National Hospice and Palliative Care Organization (NHPCO) at http://www.nhpco.org. If the family is not computer literate, advise them to get books about the grieving process from the librarian at their local Public Library branch or from the Elisabeth Kübler-Ross Foundation in Scottsdale, AZ. If the family wants you to continue contact with them after the death occurs, be cautious. Ensure contact is appropriate and does not consume your free time.

<u>CNA and bereavement period</u>

The interdisciplinary team develops a *therapeutic bond* with the family during the peri-death period. After the death occurs, it takes time for family members to let go of their relationships with the staff. Honor the emotions of the family if they want you to attend memorial services with other team members, and if you are able to do so without undue stress. You may be required to cover your head, remove your shoes, wear certain colors, or avoid opposite-sex participants. Often, attendance at services comforts the family and honors the memory of their loved one. However, be aware that some religions restrict attendance at services, and do not be insulted if you are not invited. For example, some Muslims strongly discourage women from attending burials. If the family progresses through the stages of grief as expected, they eventually are able to terminate attachment with the Hospice and Palliative Care Team.

Funeral plans

The patient bonds with the CNA because of the significant amount of time they spend together. The patient trusts the CNA and often wants to discuss funeral arrangements. This may be because it is difficult for the patient to talk with family members about funeral arrangements for fear of upsetting them, or simply that the CNA is the consistent presence for the patient. Whatever the reason, the CNA should relay the patient's wishes, if given permission to do so. The CNA is in a position to facilitate open, honest communication between the patient and his or her family, but should avoid becoming embroiled in emotional family dynamics. The CNA's responsibility as a patient advocate is to communicate the patient's wishes. If the CNA is unable to communicate with family members, he or she should turn to senior members of the healthcare team for assistance.

Interdisciplinary Collaboration

Care planning

Every hospice patient has a *nursing care plan* in his or her chart, which contains: The nursing assessment; diagnosis; risks; suspected problems; goals with dates; interventions; and expected outcomes. The nursing care plan tells the CNA about the *frequency* for performing care, for example: Position changes; ambulation; exercises; vital signs; and feeding. The care plan is a working document that the RN updates to reflect the patient's changing care needs. The CNA documents changes in the patient's condition and responses to treatment in the care plan. The care plan is separate from the *doctor's orders*, which focus on medical and surgical treatments, and medications. The CNA contributes significantly to the care plan by incorporating the likes and dislikes of the patient that impact care. The care plan is one of the most important documents in the patient record, and the CNA should participate in its development.

Multidisciplinary team members

The effective CNA knows the patient's likes and dislikes, daily pattern, and culture. This knowledge is vital for developing a humane, holistic care plan. The CNA can suggest timing care to avoid significant patient fatigue and pain. The primary goal of care is to meet the patient's needs. The secondary goal of care is to help the family. All disciplines contribute to the care plan, with everyone on the team inputting expertise and experience of equal value to minimize gaps and prevent duplication. The CNA is a key patient advocate, who brings to the team the issues that most concern the patient and family. Your team likely uses a preprinted care plan based on typical patients, which they then individualize for your patient. Software care plans save time, because the NANDA, NIC & NOC labels are already programmed. You can obtain care plans from Mosby and http://www.ltcsbooks.com. The care plan is sometimes abbreviated POC (plan of care).

Encouraging family participation

The role of the CNA is to assist and provide patient care according to the nursing care plan. Care must meet the needs of the patient and strive to be in accordance with family wishes. You can find the international standards for hospice and palliative care at http://www.hospicecare.com/standards/. Some patients participate fully in their own care, while others prefer to allow the CNA and interdisciplinary team to provide care without assistance. This passivity is often distressing for the CNA, the patient's family and all members of the interdisciplinary team. The CNA is familiar and in a position to encourage the patient and family to participate in care. Some patients prefer to have family members only provide care, which can exhaust the family. Explain to your patient that no one should feel pressured to do something he or she finds uncomfortable, and that everyone needs a break sometimes. Train family caregivers to provide correct care while using good body mechanics.

Team meetings

A 2007 study by Drs. Yeatts and Cready showed that CNAs who participate at team meetings feel empowered, give better performance, have greater self-esteem, more job satisfaction, and are less likely to be absent or quit. As a frontline worker who spends the most time with the patient and family, the CNA should contribute to developing the care plan at team meetings. The CNA may have information regarding the likes and dislikes of a patient, and often hears concerns raised by the patient or family before the rest of the staff. The team meeting is a forum for open discussion. All members of the healthcare team should be allowed an opportunity to voice concerns and comment on what aspects of the plan of care (POC) are working well. The CNA should make respectful suggestions for improving care. Your hospice may allow family members and friends who are caregivers to attend team meetings. The drawbacks of team meetings are that they take time away from patient care and require scheduling changes.

Working with Registered Nurse

The CNA is obligated to follow the care plan as directed, and report any changes or deviation from the plan to the Registered Nurse. The nursing care plan is a legal document in the patient record and can be subpoenaed to court. Use a black or dark blue pen when you write in it — never use pencil. The nursing care plan is intended to be reviewed and revised as the patient's condition changes. *All* members of the team collaborate to develop the care plan to reflect the actual needs of the patient, and keep it current. The CNA can detect and determine when changes in clinical status or family dynamics have occurred that necessitate a change in the care plan, because the CNA spends the most time with the patient. The CNA must report these changes to the Registered Nurse immediately, and work to develop a new care plan. Look for changes in the care plan at the start of your shift.

Communicating family goals

The CNA often learns the innermost thoughts and feelings of both the patient and family members through spending extensive time in the sick room. Other team members spend very limited time there, so the patient and family are less likely to hold open discussions around them. The CNA is obligated to seek the best way to meet the needs of the patient and family. Bring the family's issues, concerns or goals to the attention of the interdisciplinary team during team meetings. If the issue is dangerous or pressing, do not wait for a team meeting — notify the RN immediately. If you are uncomfortable for any reason at a team meeting, then seek out individual members of the interdisciplinary team for a private discussion afterwards. Remember that your patient and family have very limited time remaining together. Bring the patient's and family's goals and wishes up for discussion to be certain those needs are met as soon as possible.

Recognizing unwitnessed death

The CNA may find the unattended patient dead. The CNA is responsible for recognizing the signs and symptoms of unwitnessed death. They are:

- Livor mortis (reddish-blue staining in the lowest body parts, as gravity draws blood downwards)
- Algor mortis (cooling of the body by 1°F per hour until it reaches room temperature)
- Rigor mortis (stiffening of the body 2—4 hours after death, which disappears after 3—4 days)
- Blood clotting
- Putrefaction (rotting from bacteria and enzymes in the intestines)

The CNA is most sensitive to these changes because he or she is familiar with the patient's body and knows the patient's usual patterns. Report these changes to the Registered Nurse if you are in a hospice or the doctor if you are in a patient's home. They can pronounce death. A CNA is not legally allowed to pronounce death.

Support during changes

All members of the team provide support to the patient and family as the patient's condition worsens and care is increased, or if the physical location of the patient must change. The homecare patient may be moved to an in-patient hospice, a long term care facility, or hospital. The staff may be entirely unfamiliar to the stressed family. Give a verbal report to the new CNA, if possible. Ensure that an up-to-date copy of the patient's chart accompanies him or her to the new facility. Ensure the patient and family receives the emotional support they require, which allows them to have a positive Hospice and Palliative Care experience. Understand that moving from one level of care to another is distressing for the patient and family— even if they were educated beforehand — because it signals death is closer. If the family and patient confide in you, it is your responsibility to ensure their needs are known and met.

Grieving families progress through the Hospice and Palliative Care experience as a unit and also as individuals. Their individual experiences may be a source of stress for the family as a whole. Family dynamics change, for example, when a breadwinner dies or a teenager wants independence and acts out. The healthcare team must recognize changes in the pecking order, and assist the family through them. The CNA will probably notice the change in family dynamics first, since the CNA is the member of the team who spends the most time with the patient and family. When the CNA notes a change, he or she should alert the healthcare team so appropriate interventions can be developed and implemented. External resources that

may be needed include: Attorneys and Legal Aid workers; Children's Aid or youth workers; Social Services; Public Health; financial planners; emergency housing services; and employment counselors.

Reviewing a death

The interdisciplinary healthcare team holds a debriefing meeting after the patient's death. CNAs and RNs are frontline workers who experience cumulative loss when many patients die, and suffer burnout if they do not receive support from all team members. The CNA has an obligation to participate fully in the team debriefing. The team leader outlines the patient's course of care. The team lists which interventions worked well, and discusses how care could be improved for the next patient. Your clients are different individuals, but what you learned in this particular case can be applied to another. In the same way, the makeup of the interdisciplinary team varies from patient to patient. Take advantage of each unique situation to learn new methods of caring for patients from each specialist on your team. Share your skill and knowledge with other team members. Your team may decide they need to contact educators, the Ethics Committee, and the Risk Manager to provide guidance about personal and institutional liability.

Ethics, Roles and Responsibilities

Identifying ethical issues

Death brings with it significant emotional burdens and raises ethical issues. Most hospices and hospitals have an Ethics Committee led by a bioethicist. The CNA must be familiar with the facility's Code of Ethics and Patients' Rights. The CNA must have insight into his or her own perceptions about death and dying. For example, when the patient starts Cheyne-Stokes breathing, do you emotionally disengage and avoid touching your patient? The CNA must tolerate multiculturalism and other religions and belief systems. For example, a Japanese Zen Buddhist accepts suicide and euthanasia, but an Irish Catholic is prohibited from both. The CNA must gain a strong understanding of the patient's personal ethics, culture, and spiritual belief system as they relate to assisted suicide, prolonging life with feeding tubes and blood transfusions, or where palliative care should be delivered. If the patient has an ethical issue, the CNA must report it to the Registered Nurse.

Reporting issues to team

Hospice and palliative care workers have a high incidence of ethical dilemmas. CNAs develop relationships with dying patients and their families because CNAs work in the patient's intimate space. CNAs are often included in family discussions surrounding difficult issues and are asked for ethical opinions when a decision must be made. *The proper forum for ethical discussions for the CNA is with the members of the interdisciplinary team, who will refer it to the Ethics Committee if necessary.* Visit http://nursingassistants.net for advice about keeping a professional distance and legal issues. Ethical issues generally include making a choice in a situation where there is no clear right or wrong answer. Often, the issues at the heart of

the matter provoke significant emotional responses from the patient and family. CNAs must remain objective and not interfere with the patient and family.

Maintaining boundaries

Patients often develop *transference* with their caregivers, meaning they unconsciously transfer feelings from other relationships to the staff. The demented patient with transference may refuse care from anyone except a beloved CNA. The CNA with transference becomes emotionally involved with the family and develops inappropriate relationships. The CNA who is overly attached to one patient may refuse to float, or may change the schedule to be assigned to that special patient, or may short change other patients and concentrate on the favorite patient. CNAs should not become involved beyond the scope of their practice. Losing objectivity means you cannot chart the patient's progress properly, and too many resources may be allocated to the favorite patient unfairly. The CNA is in a more powerful position than the patient and family, and must not abuse that power. Turn to the psychologist on your interdisciplinary team for assistance if you feel you crossed a professional boundary.

The CNA must behave professionally and maintain boundaries with patients and their families. The experience of death and dying is emotionally complex. The CNA must not lose sight of professional obligations and begin to feel more like a friend to the patient and family than a healthcare professional. It is the responsibility of the CNA to be aware of this possibility and to seek guidance from the hospice program's psychologist, or the person on the interdisciplinary team who is designated to deal with transference. Inappropriate behaviors include:

- Spending off-duty time with the patient/family
- Keeping secrets with the patient/family or spying for the patient/family
- Becoming defensive when another team member questions your relationship with the family
- Giving and receiving gifts with the patient/family
- Flirting or having sex with the patient/family
- Siding with a patient against the staff or family
- Feeling possessive about a patient

Work-related conflicts

The Hospice and Palliative Care setting is an emotional situation. Work-related conflicts may arise within the health care team. For example:

- The CNA who favors a patient may change the work schedule
- Another member of the interdisciplinary team may disregard the CNA's comments at a team meeting
- The CNA may strongly advocate that a family be allowed to perform a religious ceremony that is against the facility's regulations and would upset other patients

It is the responsibility of all members of the interdisciplinary healthcare team to work together collaboratively and attempt to avoid conflicts. When conflicts appear, all members of the team are obligated to seek resolution to provide excellent care. Most Hospice and Palliative Care programs have a mediator in Human Resources, and educators provide conflict resolution classes. The clients are experiencing an intensely emotional situation. All team members must present themselves with confidence and behave professionally so the clients can focus on their remaining time together, and not on a dysfunctional team.

Maintaining documentation

The medical record of the Hospice and Palliative Care patient is a legal document that captures the activities and clinical care of the patient. It can be subpoenaed to court if a lawsuit is filed. All members of the interdisciplinary healthcare team must maintain accurate documentation throughout a patient's stay. Follow your program and state regulations, rules and guidelines regarding documentation. You must have full understanding of your role and responsibilities regarding documentation. Ask your Nurse Manager or union steward for a copy of your job description, which outlines how you document. CNAs receive general education surrounding documentation when in training and specialized training from their facility or agency. If you have questions or do not understand your role in documentation, it is your responsibility to obtain clarification from the designated person on your team or an educator. Obtain specifics through your state's Board of Nursing.

Reporting risks

All members of the interdisciplinary healthcare team recognize the importance of identifying and reporting risks to the safety of their patient. However, many team members fail to safeguard their own personal safety. Remember that the bereaved family is intensely emotional and may commit violence. Tactfully observe their cultural and spiritual background, because transgressing these belief systems will impact their behavior. Human Resources and the Security Manager will provide education regarding personal safety. Report personal threats or threats to another team member to Security, your Nurse Manager or team leader. If you are unsatisfied with their response, do not hesitate to contact the police.

Mentor for new staff

One of the responsibilities of healthcare professionals is the education and training of new staff and students. As healthcare professionals mature in their specialty, it is vital to the growth of the profession that others are attracted into the field. Professional CNAs act as mentors and preceptors, and this is usually an unpaid position, or carries a small stipend. The mentor shares personal dedication, passion and commitment with newcomers entering the facility. Your facility will require students to have malpractice insurance. Document mentoring and preceptorship on your résumé, as it may help convince your Nurse Manager that you are worthy of promotion. Most Hospice and Palliative Care programs offer CNAs mentoring classes and training materials.

Committee participation

One of the most important functions of the members of the interdisciplinary healthcare team is to provide educational opportunities within their area of expertise. These educational sessions serve to further the field of practice and ultimately improve the care provided to Hospice and Palliative Care patients and their families. In order for programs to function and grow, there must be staff willing to work together to facilitate this growth. The CNA can participate within program, facility or agency, or at the state level. Contribute to the education of others in your area of expertise. It improves practice and enhances patient care. Participating in committees boosts the reputation of CNAs and may gain your program additional funding.

Continuing education

Advances in healthcare are happening rapidly. Research in biology, chemistry, medicine, nursing and ethics are continually challenging the healthcare industry to revise best practices. You may be asked to trial these practice changes or collect study data. Nursing research is leading the way toward new patient care delivery models. Since the CNA is on the front line of patient care, it is imperative that you be up-to-date with the latest information. Patients are entitled to receive state-of-the-art care. Most Hospice and Palliative Care programs provide free educational opportunities for all members of the interdisciplinary team that focus on the most recent developments in the field. The CNA is required to know best practices and how to find them in the policies & procedure manual. Education updates form part of your annual performance evaluation.

Professional organizations

All professions have organizations that provide discussion forums and educational opportunities related to their specialty. Remain up-to-date with the latest research and changes in practice. Join a citizens' group like the National Coalition for Nursing Home Reform at http://www.nccnhr.org, or a professional organization for CNAs, like the National Association for Health Care Assistants at http://www.nahcacares.org. If you prefer to work with certain types of patients, join an association that deals with that group, such as UNAIDS or Cystic Fibrosis Worldwide. A politically active CNA brings to the team additional resources for the patient, adds value to the team, and can provide educational opportunities for the facility. Most state nursing associations include a CNA subdivision. It is the responsibility of all healthcare professionals to work to advance their practice in order to deliver excellent patient care.

Peer reviews

Annual performance evaluation is required in most organizations. Some facilities conduct performance evaluations by having the supervisor of the CNA assess and evaluate the CNA. Others incorporate a peer review process into the evaluation. Participation in a peer review is a responsibility the CNA should accept as a professional. The evaluation process should be conducted fairly and honestly, without regard to personal friendships. Your Human Resources Department will offer training regarding the peer review process. Before actively participating in a peer review, have a clear understanding of your employer's expectations for you as a reviewer and the parameters of the review. If you do not believe you can participate objectively for any reason, alert your supervisor and union steward and decline participation.

Quality Improvement activities

Your facility will designate a Quality Assurance (QA) officer or CPHQ. Quality improvement activities in the field of Hospice and Palliative Care are directed at patient care and minimizing staff injuries. QA activities can take on many forms:

- Accreditation to keep your facility's operating license
- Active research that brings about changes in patient care
- Feedback from patients and their families that brings a change in practice
- New federal and state licensing regulations and laws
- Risk Management changes in response to lawsuits

Regardless of the nature of the quality improvement activities, the CNA is required to participate fully as a member of the interdisciplinary healthcare team. This means helping the QA officer to gather data, test theories, and disseminate findings. QA uses the scientific method. A CNA who wants to move into a supervisor's role must learn about QA.

Practice Test

Practice Test

1. When using music therapy to help a patient relax, the most important criterion is
    a. Genre of music.
    b. Patient preference.
    c. Delivery system.
    d. Rhythm and beat.

2. Which type of precautions require that the nurse assistant wear a mask while caring for the patient, that the patient be separated from other patients by at least 3 feet with a curtain separating them, and that a patient mask be used during transport?
    a. Standard
    b. Contact
    c. Airborne
    d. Droplet

3. A dying patient has taken no fluids for 24 hours. Which measure is most appropriate to alleviate discomfort from dehydration?
    a. Providing mouth care and moistening mucous membranes.
    b. Administering intravenous fluids.
    c. Placing ice chips in the patient's mouth.
    d. Encouraging sips of fluid.

4. A patient is nearing death and has started to develop a pressure area on the sacral area but moans loudly and is resistive when the nurse assistant tries to turn him. The best action is to
    a. Turn the patient frequently to prevent further skin deterioration.
    b. Allow the patient to lie undisturbed as much as possible.
    c. Ask the nurse to increase pain medication so that the patient can be turned.
    d. Ask to transfer the patient to a bed with an alternating pressure mattress.

5. The nurse assistant is in the room and attending the immediate and extended family of a dying infant during the death vigil. The mother is very upset and angry with the doctor for not saving her child. The most appropriate action for the nurse assistant is
    a. Reassure the family that the child's suffering will soon be over.
    b. Sit quietly and interact with family if they desire.
    c. Explain to the mother that the doctor is not to blame.
    d. Hug the mother to provide comfort.

6. When a Buddhist patient dies, the family asks that no one touch the body for at least 4 hours. The reason for this is probably because the family
    a. Needs time to come to terms with the patient's death.
    b. Believes that the soul stays with the body after death and needs time to leave in peace.
    c. Wants time to pray for the patient's soul.
    d. Wants time to wash and prepare the body.

7. A patient with end-stage liver disease has had repeat paracenteses to relieve dyspnea. What measure is routinely done to assess the degree of ascites?
    a. Vital signs.
    b. Blood tests.
    c. Waist and hip circumference.
    d. Weight and waist circumference.

8. A common respiratory pattern found in dying patients is
    a. Cheyne-Stokes respirations.
    b. Kussmaul respirations.
    c. Tachypnea.
    d. Bradypnea.

9. A common sign of impending death is
    a. Increased body temperature
    b. Pinpoint pupils.
    c. Waxy pallor.
    d. Rapid heartbeat.

10. The most important criterion for determining the degree of a patient's pain is
    a. Physical indication, such as grimacing or guarding.
    b. Moaning.
    c. Patient report.
    d. Patient history.

11. After a patient receives morphine for pain, which of the following symptoms is most cause for concern?
    a. Patient develops moderate myoclonus (twitching).
    b. Patient's respirations slow from 20 to 16 per minute.
    c. Patient falls into a deep sleep.
    d. Patient appears lethargic.

12. Bereavement is
    a. A normal response to loss.
    b. The public expression of grief.
    c. Change of mood and feeling of sadness.
    d. The time period of mourning.

13. The nurse assistant enters a patient's room after he talks to the doctor and finds the patient shaking and distraught. Which is the best response?
    a. "What's wrong?"
    b. "Do you want me to call your family?"
    c. "You are shaking and seem worried."
    d. "You don't need to worry. Everything will be all right."

14. What is the minimal urinary output per hour expected for an adult patient?
    a. 20 mL
    b. 30 mL
    c. 40 mL
    d. 50 mL

15. The supervising nurse asks the nurse assistant to check a patient's gastrostomy tube to see if it has migrated, but the nurse assistant is unsure what this means. The nurse assistant should
    a. Immediately inform the nurse she doesn't know how to do this.
    b. Ask another nurse assistant to help.
    c. Check the gastrostomy tube to see if it looks all right.
    d. Check the procedure manual.

16. A 48-year-old female patient has terminal ovarian cancer but states she believes her doctor has misdiagnosed her and wants to see a different doctor. Which stage of Elisabeth Kübler-Ross's stages of grief (death and dying) is she likely experiencing?
    a. Anger.
    b. Denial.
    c. Depression.
    d. Bargaining.

17. Which of the following is part of formal closure activities after a patient dies?
    a. Sending a gift to the surviving family member.
    b. Sending a card of condolences.
    c. Assisting family to make funeral arrangements.
    d. Establishing an ongoing long-term relationship.

18. A hospice patient nearing death should be offered food and fluids until
    a. The patient loses consciousness.
    b. The patient stops showing interest.
    c. The patient begins artificial feeding and hydration.
    d. The patient becomes lethargic, sleeping much of the time.

19. A patient has stopped eating most sources of protein because of unrelieved nausea and is rapidly losing muscle mass. A good way to increase protein and caloric intake is to
    a. Add eggs and/or protein powder to foods the patient can tolerate.
    b. Provide meat at every meal and insist the patient eat some.
    c. Tell the patient how important protein is in his/her diet.
    d. Encourage plant-based proteins, such as beans.

20. Which of the follow symptoms occurs in almost all terminal cancer patients at the end of life?
    a. Depression.
    b. Nausea and vomiting.
    c. Anxiety.
    d. Anorexia.

21. A patient who usually showers states she is too fatigued and asks the nurse assistant to give her a partial sponge bath. The best action is to
    a. Tell the patient that she should make the effort to take a shower.
    b. Tell the patient she can take the shower later in the day.
    c. Give the patient a partial sponge bath as requested.
    d. Tell the patient that she can wait until the next day to bathe.

22. A patient receiving an opioid for pain management is having increased constipation and is undergoing bowel retraining. Which is the best time to assist the patient to sit on a toilet or commode to promote evacuation?
    a. First thing in the morning.
    b. About 20 to 30 minutes after a meal.
    c. When the patient feels an urge to defecate.
    d. Last thing before bedtime.

23. A patient nearing death has been experiencing delirium, with marked confusion and hallucinations. The patient believes the nurse assistant is her child and asks if everything is all right at home. An appropriate response is
    a. "Everything is fine at home."
    b. "You are confused about who I am."
    c. "I am your nurse assistant, John Smith."
    d. "I'm not your child."

24. A patient had always been active in many sports and is now chair-bound, bored, and becoming depressed. When helping the family to provide recreational activities, the nurse assistant suggests
    a. Video sport games.
    b. Books about sports.
    c. Paper puzzles, such as Sudoku and crossword puzzles.
    d. Board games.

25. A patient dying of lung cancer is very dyspneic. The head of the bed is elevated to 45° and he is receiving oxygen at 4 L/min. Which of the following interventions is best to help the patient feel less anxious about the shortness of breath?
    a. Playing soft music.
    b. Increasing fluid intake.
    c. Directing the airflow of an electric fan toward the patient's face.
    d. Sitting the patient upright (at 90°) in bed.

26. A patient needs a walker to ambulate. For maximum support, the height of the walker should be adjusted so the individual's elbows are bent at
    a. 0 to 5 degrees.
    b. 5 to 10 degrees.
    c. 10 to 20 degrees.
    d. 20 to 30 degrees.

27. When conducting range of motion (ROM) exercises, the sequence should be
    a. From the head down.
    b. From the bottom up.
    c. Right side first and then left side.
    d. From the head to the waist and then the feet to the hips.

28. A hospitalized patient asks the nurse assistant to stop by his house to pick up his mail and offers $20 to pay for gas and time spent. The nurse assistant should
    a. Get the mail but refuse the money.
    b. Offer to help the patient make other arrangements for someone to pick up his mail.
    c. Get the mail and accept the money with thanks.
    d. Get the mail and charge only for mileage.

29. A patient has had persistent nausea and vomiting despite receiving medication to control her symptoms. Which of the following measures may provide some relief?
    a. Increasing fluid intake with foods.
    b. Serving foods warm to hot.
    c. Asking the patient to lie flat after eating.
    d. Asking the patient do deep breathing and controlled swallowing.

30. As a patient nears death, an audible gurgling is heard as the patient breathes. The best way to explain this to the family is
    a. "Congestion in the throat and lungs occurs as fluids accumulate."
    b. "These are the death rattles."
    c. "He is starting to drown in his own body fluids."
    d. "This sounds bad, but it's perfectly normal."

31. A patient in a shared room enjoys listening to music on a small radio that his son brought to him, but the patient in the adjoining bed complains that the music prevents him from resting. The best solution is for the nurse assistant to

    a. Tell the patient with the radio that he cannot use it.
    b. Ask the patient with the radio to get earphones.
    c. Ask the patient who is disturbed to use earplugs.
    d. Ask the supervisor if one patient can be moved to another room.

32. In documenting a patient's condition, which of the following is an objective statement?
    a. "Patient seems very sleepy."
    b. "Patient complains he is not getting enough rest at night."
    c. "Patient slept after lunch from 1 to 4 PM."
    d. "The patient's pain medication is making him too sleepy."

33. A fever that rises and falls but never falls below 99.6°F/37.6°C would be described as
    a. Remittent.
    b. Relapsing.
    c. Intermittent.
    d. Continuous.

34. A patient with cognitive impairment and metastatic colon cancer is receiving pain medication around the clock, but the nurse assistant notes that the patient has short periods of hyperventilation, cries out frequently, is lying rigidly with fists clenched, and is increasingly combative. The nurse assistant should suspect
    a. Inadequate pain control.
    b. Excess sedation from pain medication.
    c. Side effects of pain medication.
    d. Increasing dementia.

35. A patient's husband is sneezing and coughing but states he has seasonal hay fever and asthma and is not infectious. The nurse assistant should advise the husband that he
    a. Needs to take no extra precautions since he is not infectious.
    b. Cannot visit until all symptoms have subsided.
    c. Could be spreading germs.
    d. Must follow standard precautions for respiratory hygiene/cough etiquette.

36. A nurse assistant caring for a confused patient in his home discovers that he has a loaded gun under his pillow. The nurse assistant should
    a. Ask the patient to put the gun in a safer place.
    b. Leave as soon as possible and notify a supervisor.
    c. Place the gun in another room.
    d. Notify the police.

37. When caring for a hospitalized patient with advanced cancer and intractable pain, the nurse assistant discovers that the patient has hidden 12 doses of a narcotic pain pill in a candy container in her bedside stand. The nurse assistant should

    a. Ask the patient why she has hidden the pills.

    b. Advise the patient that the nurse assistant must ring for a supervising nurse and report the findings.

    c. Ignore the finding.

    d. Call the patient's family and report the finding.

38. The nurse assistant conducts a written survey of a group of 15 nurse assistants regarding work conditions but receives only 5 responses. However, all 5 are unhappy with work conditions. Based on this sample, the researcher must conclude that

    a. These 5 represent the feelings of the entire group of 15.

    b. These 5 do not represent the feelings of the entire group of 15.

    c. These findings apply to the 5 respondents only.

    d. No interpretation is possible.

39. During a team meeting, the team leader reports that Mrs. Smith is responding well to treatment and is in good spirits, but the nurse assistant had found Mrs. Smith in her bathroom depressed and crying for the last 2 days and reported her observations. The nurse assistant should

    a. Take the team leader aside later and again report her findings.

    b. Report her observation during the team meeting.

    c. Ask why her reports have been ignored.

    d. Report the team leader to a supervisor.

40. As a patient is nearing death, the patient's daughter states that she would like to do something to help care for her mother but she is unsure what to do. The nurse assistant should

    a. Tell the daughter that her presence is enough.

    b. Tell the daughter her help isn't needed.

    c. Tell the daughter to hold her mother's hand and talk to her.

    d. Show the daughter how to do simple procedures, such as mouth care.

41. A patient who is nearing death tells the nurse assistant that her family has not yet arrived, and she regrets that she not talked to them more openly. The best response is

    a. "You can tell me what you'd like them to know about you, and I'll write it down for you."

    b. "I'm sure your family loves you."

    c. "Most people don't say all that they should."

    d. "Your family will be here soon."

42. A dying patient repeatedly calls out "Mama" and picks at her bedclothes. The son asks what he should do. The nurse assistant should advise him to
    a. Go home, as the patient no longer knows he is there.
    b. Orient the patient by reminding her that he is her son.
    c. Talk softly to her and hold her hand or touch her to provide comfort.
    d. Tell the patient, "Your mama is here."

43. A gay man dying of HIV/AIDS asks that his parents, who have come to the hospice begging to see him, not be allowed into his room because they have refused to accept his lifestyle and his partner. The best action for the nurse assistant is to
    a. Urge the man to reconsider.
    b. Allow the parents into the room.
    c. Tell the parents their son does not want to see them.
    d. Tell the parents they can leave a message for their son but cannot visit him.

44. According to the patient's care plan, he is at risk of falls because of confusion. Which therapeutic intervention should the nurse assistant expect to carry out?
    a. Leave all side rails up.
    b. Apply a body restraint.
    c. Leave all overhead lights in the room on at night.
    d. Apply a motion sensor.

45. When addressing a patient who is hearing impaired but not deaf, the best approach is to
    a. Speak loudly.
    b. Use simplified language.
    c. Speak slowly and clearly, facing the person.
    d. Communicate through writing only.

46. If participating in peer review, the nursing assistant would be responsible for evaluating
    a. All team members.
    b. Other nursing assistants.
    c. Any medical staff.
    d. Patients.

47. The nursing assistant notes that a newly admitted, anxious elderly patient has bilateral bruises on her trunk and limbs in several stages of healing, including about her wrists, and has very poor physical and dental hygiene. During the care plan conference, the nursing assistant should express concerns about possible
    a. Abuse and neglect.
    b. Falls.
    c. Bleeding disorder.
    d. Low income.

48. When assisting a patient to ambulate, the nurse assistant notes that the patient develops labored breathing and pulse rate increases 40 bpm over base rate during ambulation. This suggests
    a. Normal changes related to exercise.
    b. General fatigue.
    c. Heart attack.
    d. Activity intolerance.

49. In helping a patient who is facing a terminal disease reframe hope, which is the most useful statement?
    a. "You still have time left."
    b. "Your faith is strong, and that will help you."
    c. "What is most important to you?"
    d. "We will be there to help you."

50. An hour after a patient dies, her daughter remains at the bedside crying, and the patient's body has not yet been prepared for transfer to the funeral home. The best action of the nurse assistant is
    a. Tell the daughter that she must leave.
    b. Remind the daughter that the attendants from the funeral home will arrive soon.
    c. Ask the daughter how much longer she wants to stay.
    d. Ask the daughter if she would like to help prepare her mother's body.

Answers and Explanations

1. B: Music therapy should be tailored to the patient's preference, and this may vary from time to time. For example, a patient may prefer upbeat music during the daytime and quieter music in the evening. While soft classical music is a good general choice, some patients may prefer other genres. Some patients may favor music related to their cultures. The delivery system may vary. In a single room, a radio or music player may be placed by the bed, but in a shared room, the volume should be turned down or the patient fitted with small earphones.

2. D: Droplet. Transmission-based precautions include:

Contact	Use personal protective equipment (PPE), including gown and gloves, for all contacts with the patient or patient's immediate environment. Maintain patient in private room or > 3 feet away from other patients.
Droplet	Use mask while caring for the patient. Maintain patient in a private room or > 3 feet away from other patients with curtain separating them. Use patient mask if transporting patient from one area to another.
Airborne	Place patient in an airborne infection isolation room. Use $\geq$ N95 respirators (or masks) while caring for patient.

3. A: Patients normally stop taking fluids as they near death, resulting in dehydration and drying of the mucous membranes of the mouth. Frequent mouth care and moistening of the mucous membranes can alleviate mouth discomfort. Mouth care includes cleaning with soft toothbrush or sponge swabs, rinsing the mouth with water, misting with a spray bottle, or placing loose damp gauze over the patient's mouth. Lips should be lubricated to prevent cracking. The mouth may be swabbed with artificial saliva, such as *Salivart*.

4. B: When a patient is nearing death, the most important consideration is comfort, even if this means that some routine patient care, such as turning the patient, must be set aside. The patient should be allowed to lie undisturbed as much as possible. Pain medication is usually decreased as a patient nears death, and increasing the medication may result in increased adverse effects. The process of transferring a patient to another bed may cause discomfort and distress.

5. C: During the death vigil, the nurse assistant should stay with the family and sit quietly, allowing them to talk, cry, or interact if they desire. Other guidelines include:
Avoid platitudes, such as "His suffering will be over soon."
Avoid judgmental reactions to what family members say or do. Realize that anger, fear, guilt, and irrational behavior are normal responses to acute grief and stress.

Show caring by touching the patient and encouraging family to do the same. Note: Touching hands, arms, or shoulders of family members can provide comfort, but follow clues of the family and avoid hugging, which may be misconstrued.
Provide referrals to support groups if available.

6. B: Because part of Buddhist belief is that the soul stays with the body for some time after death, family members may wish to leave the deceased undisturbed for a period of time to allow the soul time to leave the body in peace. Buddhists believe that the soul experiences multiple lifetimes to learn necessary lessons and that actions in a previous lifetime influence the current life, including illnesses, and that death is a natural part of the transition from one life to another.

7. D: Ascites is routinely assessed by taking daily weight and measuring the waist circumference. Ascites is an accumulation of fluid in the peritoneal cavity, resulting in pressure on the diaphragm and preventing adequate respirations, so patients often become very short of breath. Small amount of ascites may not be obvious, but as fluid is retained, weight increases and the abdominal girth expands, with the abdomen often markedly protuberant. Paracentesis can provide temporary relief, but the fluid accumulates again. Fluid restriction, diuretics, and sodium restriction may help slow the accumulation.

8. A: Cheyne-Stokes respirations are commonly found in dying patients. About three-quarters of those dying experience terminal dyspnea. As the lungs become less effective and more congested, gas exchange is poor, and carbon dioxide levels increase. This increase usually triggers respiration, but as brain function decreases, this function is impaired, so respirations may deepen and then become more shallow and irregular with periods of apnea that may last for up to a minute in a repeating cycle.

9. B: As death approaches, body temperature begins to drop slowly and the skin takes on a waxy pallor. Pupils at death become fixed and dilated. Other indications include a lack of heartbeat and respirations. The patient does not respond to stimuli. As the muscles relax, the patient may be incontinent of urine and/or feces. The dying process is generally not immediate, and these changes may not occur sequentially. Patients, for example, may stop breathing and then start again or gasp a time or two before breathing stops completely.

10. C: Patient report is the most important criterion for determining the degree of a patient's pain. People may perceive and express pain very differently, so unless drug-seeking or attention-seeking behavior can be established, the nurse assistant should accept that the patient's pain is as reported. Some cultures encourage outward expressions of pain while others do not. Various pain scales may be used, depending on the age and cognitive ability of the patient. The most commonly used scale for adolescents and adults is the 1 to 10 scale.

11. A: Myoclonus (twitching) is common after opioid administration and mild twitching is usually not of major concern, but moderate or more pronounced myoclonus may result in seizures. The medication dosage may need to be decreased to control the myoclonus, or

two or three different medications should be given in rotation. Respirations of 16 to 20 are both in the range of normal. Lethargy and sleeping often occur with opioids because of their sedative effects and are not cause for concern if the patient is otherwise stable.

12. D: Bereavement is the time period of mourning. This time period varies but may extend to a year or even longer. Grief is a normal response to loss while mourning is the public expression of grief. The three types of grief are acute, anticipatory, and chronic. Chronic grief poses a serious risk to people and should be considered depression and treated with antidepressants, psychological evaluation, and counselling. Depression is characterized by changes in mood and feelings of sadness.

13. C: "You are shaking and seem worried" acknowledges what is true and evident and leaves an opening for the patient to discuss his feelings if he wants to. "What's wrong?" requires a direct response the patient may not feel like giving. "Do you want me to call your family" does not deal with the patient's anxiety and is an escape for the nurse assistant. "You don't need to worry. Everything will be all right" is a platitude that has little meaning and may not, in fact, be true.

14. B: The minimal urinary output for an adult patient is 30 mL/h, although this level cannot be sustained for long periods, as a more normal output is 40 to 60 mL/h. Minimal output for an infant or child is 0.5 mL/kg/h. Output < 30 mL/h may signal renal damage. Urinary output is influenced not only by renal status but also by hydration and medications. Vasoconstrictive medications may reduce urinary output. Patients may have low output after surgery and then diuresis as their systems clear anesthetic drugs and other medications.

15. A: The nurse assistant should immediately inform the nurse that she doesn't know how to do this. The nurse who delegates remains accountable for patient outcomes and for supervision of the person to whom the task was delegated. Delegation should be done in a manner that reduces liability by providing adequate communication. This includes specific directions about the task, including what needs to be done, when, and for how long. Expectations related to consultation, reporting, and completion of tasks should be clearly defined. The nurse should be available to assist if necessary.

16. D: The patient is experiencing the stage of bargaining, during which the patient/family may change doctors in an effort to change the outcome. People grieve individually and may not go through all stages, but most go through at least 2 stages. Kübler-Ross's 5 stages of grief include:
Denial: disbelieving, confused, stunned, detached, repeating questions.
Anger: directed inward (self-blame) or outward.
Bargaining: if/then thinking. (If I go to church, then I will heal.) Trying to find a different outcome.
Depression: Sad, withdrawn, tearful, crying but beginning to accept loss.
Acceptance: Resolution and acceptance.

17. B: Telephoning family members and/or sending a card or message of condolences, not a gift, is an appropriate closure activity. Assisting the family to make funeral arrangements is outside of the expected formal closure activities and responsibilities of the nursing assistant. However, making a final visit with the family after a patient's death can help family find closure. In some cases, family members may want to establish long-term relationships with health care providers, but this can establish a dependent relationship that may prove detrimental.

18. B: The patient should be offered food and fluids as long as the patient shows any interest. At some point, the patient no longer wants food or fluid or derives any pleasure from them, even though the patient may still be conscious. Lethargy does not warrant withholding food and fluids if the patient can be easily aroused from sleep. Artificial feeding and hydration are not recommended for patients who are dying because it extends suffering, although some patients and their families may choose this option.

19. A: Eggs and/or protein powder can be added to many foods to increase protein intake. For example, custards can be prepared with double or triple the usual number of eggs without affecting palatability. People with nausea often avoid meat products and those that can cause gas, such as beans. Simply telling patients to eat better is not usually enough to overcome the negative effects of nausea on diet. Chilled dietary supplement drinks, such as *Ensure*, may be added to the diet if the patient can tolerate them.

20. D: Almost all patients with terminal cancer experience anorexia while about half have nausea and vomiting, one-quarter to one-half have anxiety, and one-quarter to three-quarters have depression. Managing anorexia includes lifting dietary restrictions, supplementing food with added protein and calories, avoiding hot food (to reduce odor), accommodating patient preferences for eating schedule and types of foods, allowing alcoholic beverages if the patient desires them, avoiding weighing the patient or stressing weight loss, and never forcing the patient to eat or drink.

21. C: The nurse assistant should comply with the patient's wishes and give her a partial sponge bath. Fatigue is very common, and patients should be allowed to rest as necessary, even if this means that they are unable to do usual activities, which may need to be modified or adjusted. For example, a patient may be able to shower with assistance using a shower chair but may feel too fatigued to stand and wash herself.

22. B: A schedule for defecation should be established, preferably at the same time each day and about 20 to 30 minutes after a meal, which stimulates the gastrocolic reflex that propels fecal material through the colon. In some cases, a stimulus may be provided to promote defecation. This may be enemas, suppositories, or laxatives in the beginning, but the goal is to decrease such use. Digital stimulation or hot drinks may be used. The patient should keep a record of stool consistency and evacuation.

23. C: Delirium is quite common in patients at the end of life, and the nurse assistant should try to help orient the patient by saying that which is true, "I am your nurse assistant, John

Smith," without pointing out that the patient is confused. Sometimes an orientation board, which may include lists of daily activities and names and pictures of family and/or caregivers, may be helpful. Reducing noise and helping the patient to relax with music or massage may decrease symptoms.

24. A: When planning recreational activities for patients, the nurse assistant should always consider patient preferences and habitual activities, even though these may need to be modified. Video sports games, such as Nintendo Wii Sports, require minimal physical input but can provide a satisfying experience of sports participation. The patient's abilities and limitations must also be considered so that the patient can successful engage in an activity. Video sports games are good for those who are chairbound because they can be played by using only the arms and hands.

25. C: Directing the airflow of an electric fan toward the patient's face may make the patient feel anxious about the shortness of breath. The patient's head is already elevated and sitting the patient straight upright in bed may compress the diaphragm and increase the dyspnea. Oxygen is usually administered at 2 to 4 L/min. If the patient is dehydrated, then increasing fluids may increase comfort but will probably not affect dyspnea because of the lung compromise associated with lung cancer.

26. D: The height of the walker should be adjusted so that the individual's elbows are bent at 20 to 30 degrees for maximum support. This allows for the arms to extend when the walker is moved forward. If the arms are bent more, the patient may fall forward or to the side as the arms cannot support the patient's weight. If the arms are straight, then the individual may not be able to move the walker forward the 18 to 24 inches that are required for a normal stride.

27. A: ROM exercises should be done in sequence from the head down. If possible, most ROM exercises should be done with the patient sitting because it is easier to attain a more normal range. Exercises of the head and neck should be done by the patient to avoid overstretching of the cervical spine. Joints should be moved through flexion, extension, rotation, supination, and pronation as appropriate for the type of joint. The best positions for exercising the hip joint are the supine position and the prone position (if tolerated).

28. B: Giving extra attention to a patient by picking up mail and accepting money for anything other than wages are both boundary violations. The nurse assistant should offer to assist the patient to make other arrangements, such as by telephoning a friend or family member. While running errands for the patient may benefit him in the short term, it can establish a relationship of increasing dependency and obligation that does not resolve the long-term needs of the patient.

29. D: Asking the patient to do deep breathing and controlled swallowing may help to control the gag/vomit reflex. Other measures include serving cold or room temperature foods, restricting intake of fluids during meals, and sitting or lying with the head elevated for at least 2 hours after eating. Patients may benefit from 5 or 6 small meals per day rather

than 3 large meals. Fluids should be sipped in small amounts throughout the day rather than drinking large amounts of fluids at one time.

30. A: "Congestion in the throat and lungs occurs as fluids accumulate" explains what is happening in simple but non-frightening terms. The nurse assistant should avoid negative terms that suggest suffering, such as "drowning in his own body fluids" or "suffocating." The term "death rattles" should also be avoided. "This sounds bad, but it's perfectly normal" doesn't help explain what causes the gurgling. If gurgling is severe and distressing to the family, some medications may help to reduce the gurgling.

31. B: Since earphones are relatively inexpensive and easy to obtain, the best solution is probably to ask the patient with the radio to get earphones. The patient may be able to keep the volume lower as well, but the nurse assistant should always try to find the solution that works best for both patients when a conflict arises. When patients are very ill or dying, even a very small annoyance can cause undue distress, and many people are very sensitive to noises of all kinds, even music.

32. C: "Patient slept after lunch from 1 to 4 PM" is objective because it reports exactly what the nurse assistant observed. Subjective statements can include the patient's statement of a problem as well as any judgmental statements, such as "the patient's pain medication is making him too sleepy," or interpreting statements, such as "the patient seems very sleepy." Documentation should be as objective as possible because one's interpretation of an observation may be wrong.

33. A: Remittent: The temperature rises and falls but always stays above normal levels (98.6°F/37°C). Relapsing: The temperature decreases to normal levels and may stay there for a while (hours, days, weeks) but then increases again. Relapse may occur several times. Intermittent: Temperatures rise and fall in a regular spiking pattern. Continuous: Temperature stays at about the same range most of the time. It may decrease with medication, such as acetaminophen, but returns to the baseline after about 4 hours.

34. A: The patient is exhibiting non-verbal indications of pain. The Pain Assessment in Advanced Dementia (PAINAD) scale includes:
Respirations: Rapid and labored breathing as pain increases with short periods of hyperventilation or Cheyne-Stokes respirations.
Vocalization: Negative in speech or speaking quietly and reluctantly, may moan or groan. As pain increases, may call out, moan or groan loudly, or cry.
Facial expression: May appear sad or frightened, may frown or grimace, especially with activity.
Body language: May be tense, fidgeting, pacing, and as pain increases rigid, clenched fists, lying in fetal position, and increasingly combative.
Consolability: Less distractible or consolable.

35. D: All patients, staff, and visitors with respiratory symptoms, regardless of diagnosis, must follow standard precautions for respiratory hygiene/cough etiquette. This includes

covering the mouth with a tissue or coughing/sneezing into the sleeve of the upper arm or the elbow, avoiding the hands because the hands can easily spread germs. Soiled tissues should be discarded promptly and hands washed. People may be asked to wear masks and should maintain a distance of at least 3 feet from others.

36. B: The nurse assistant should always remove himself/herself from an unsafe situation as soon as possible and notify a supervisor. A confused patient should not have access to any dangerous weapons, and asking the patient to put the gun in a safer place increases risk to the patient and the nurse. The nurse assistant should not touch or move a dangerous weapon. Whether or not the police should be notified is an issue for the supervisor. Many people have licenses for handguns.

37. B: The nurse assistant should advise the patient that he or she must ring for a nurse to report the findings. Patients who are suicidal may hoard pills so that they can take an overdose. It is the supervising nurse's responsibility to handle medication problems and to speak with the patient to determine the reason the patient was hoarding the medications. HIPAA regulations preclude reporting any information about a patient to family members without the patient's consent.

38. C: These findings apply to the 5 respondents only. With such a small response, those in the majority may have chosen not to respond at all, so the results may be skewed toward the minority. Generally, the smaller the group size, the larger the required proportion for sampling. Thus, with 15 in the group, a sample size must be around 14 to ensure a reasonable degree of accuracy. As the size increases, the proportion decreases. For example, at 250, a sample size of 150 is adequate.

39. B: There can be many reasons why reports are overlooked or forgotten, but as an advocate for the patient, the nurse assistant should simply report her observations during the team meeting in a respectful manner so that the others on the team can discuss the problem and arrive at a plan. One of the advantages of collaborating in a team environment is that issues that may have been overlooked can be brought to the team's attention.

40. D: The nurse assistant should show the daughter how to do simple procedures, such as mouth care, because this responds to the daughter's specific request "to help with her mother's care." Family members often feel helpless as their loved ones are dying, so having tasks to do helps them to feel needed and useful and can be very rewarding. While holding her mother's hand and talking to her is also good advice, it doesn't respond to the daughter's request.

41. A: The best response is to give the patient the opportunity to do a life review: "You can tell me what you'd like them to know about you, and I'll write it down for you." A life review helps a dying patient to arrive at an acceptance of death and to make peace with those things done or neglected. Asking open-ended questions, such as "What do you remember about your childhood?" can help guide a patient through the process.

42. C: The best advice for the son is to talk softly to the mother and hold her hand or touch her to comfort her. As death nears, people often wander in and out of consciousness, and hallucinations and confusion are common. People often call out for their mothers, regardless of their age. They may mistake one family member for another, and often are restless or pick at bedclothes. The nurse assistant should explain to the son that as the brain begins to shut down, these changes in awareness are normal.

43. D: Giving the parents the opportunity to leave a message while respecting the patient's absolute right to bar them from visiting him is probably the best action. Then, it is up to the patient whether to read the message or not. Families often try to make amends before someone dies, but it is impossible for the nurse assistant to know what motivates the parents in this situation or the type of history the parents and the patient share.

44. D: A motion sensor can help to warn staff that the patient is trying to climb out of bed. Patients often fall trying to climb over bed rails, so it is usually safer to leave at least one rail down with the bed in the lowest position. Patients should not be placed in body restraints. Patients who are confused may need a somewhat darkened room to sleep, but a nightlight should be left on. All staff members should be made aware that the patient is at risk for falls. Belongings and the call bell should be kept within easy reach.

45. C: The nurse assistant should speak slowly and clearly, facing the patient, so that the patient can obtain visual cues to aid in comprehension. It is important to avoid shouting or speaking excessively loudly and to have pen and paper available in case it is needed to enhance communication. If the patient cannot understand what is said, the nurse assistant can rephrase but should avoid using extremely simplified, child-like language because hearing impairment is not associated with mental impairment. Family members may provide information about the best way to communicate with the hearing impaired.

46. B: Peer review is an intensive process in which an individual practitioner is reviewed by like practitioners, so a nursing assistant would review other nursing assistants. A ranking system is usually used to indicate compliance with standards:
Care is based on standards and typical of that provided by like practitioners.
Variance may occur in care, but outcomes are satisfactory.
Care is not consistent with that provided by like practitioners.
Variance resulted in negative outcomes.

47. A: These are indications of abuse and neglect. Abuse may be difficult to diagnose, especially if the person is cognitively impaired, but symptoms can include fearfulness, disparities in reports of injuries between patient and caregiver, evidence of old or repeated injuries, bilateral bruises in various stages of healing, poor hygiene and dental care, decubiti, malnutrition, undue concern with costs on caregiver's part, unsupportive attitude of caregiver, and caregiver's reluctance or refusal to allow patient to communicate privately with the nurse.

48. D: Labored breathing and an increased pulse rate more than 20 to 30 bpm occurring during an activity are indications of activity intolerance. Patients may also become light-headed, dizzy, and pale or diaphoretic, and systolic BP may increase >20 mm Hg or decrease >10 mm Hg. Activity intolerance can result from multiple factors, such as a chronic condition, obesity, general weakness, and debility. Activities must be geared to the patient's ability with adequate rest periods, and patients taught to recognize the signs of physical overactivity.

49. C: "What is most important to you?" helps the patient to focus on reframing hope toward an achievable goal. For some patients, this may be to remain pain free while others may want to spend time with family or complete a project. Once a patient can identify a goal or multiple goals, the nursing assistant must work with the patient and other members of the health care team to ensure that the patient's wishes are known and that a plan is made to help the patient achieve the goals.

50. D: The nurse assistant should ask the daughter if she would like to help prepare her mother's body. This is a gentle way to remind the daughter that the body must be removed, and it allows her to provide a service that may be rewarding. Many people are unfamiliar with death but would like to do something to help them find closure. These people may be unsure what to do, so the nurse assistant can provide guidance.

Secret Key #1 - Time is Your Greatest Enemy

Pace Yourself

Wear a watch. At the beginning of the test, check the time (or start a chronometer on your watch to count the minutes), and check the time after every few questions to make sure you are "on schedule."

If you are forced to speed up, do it efficiently. Usually one or more answer choices can be eliminated without too much difficulty. Above all, don't panic. Don't speed up and just begin guessing at random choices. By pacing yourself, and continually monitoring your progress against your watch, you will always know exactly how far ahead or behind you are with your available time. If you find that you are one minute behind on the test, don't skip one question without spending any time on it, just to catch back up. Take 15 fewer seconds on the next four questions, and after four questions you'll have caught back up. Once you catch back up, you can continue working each problem at your normal pace.

Furthermore, don't dwell on the problems that you were rushed on. If a problem was taking up too much time and you made a hurried guess, it must be difficult. The difficult questions are the ones you are most likely to miss anyway, so it isn't a big loss. It is better to end with more time than you need than to run out of time.

Lastly, sometimes it is beneficial to slow down if you are constantly getting ahead of time. You are always more likely to catch a careless mistake by working more slowly than quickly, and among very high-scoring test takers (those who are likely to have lots of time left over), careless errors affect the score more than mastery of material.

Secret Key #2 - Guessing is not Guesswork

You probably know that guessing is a good idea. Unlike other standardized tests, there is no penalty for getting a wrong answer. Even if you have no idea about a question, you still have a 20-25% chance of getting it right.

Most test takers do not understand the impact that proper guessing can have on their score. Unless you score extremely high, guessing will significantly contribute to your final score.

Monkeys Take the Test

What most test takers don't realize is that to insure that 20-25% chance, you have to guess randomly. If you put 20 monkeys in a room to take this test, assuming they answered once per question and behaved themselves, on average they would get 20-25% of the questions correct. Put 20 test takers in the room, and the average will be much lower among guessed questions. Why?

1. The test writers intentionally write deceptive answer choices that "look" right. A test taker has no idea about a question, so he picks the "best looking" answer, which is often wrong. The monkey has no idea what looks good and what doesn't, so it will consistently be right about 20-25% of the time.

2. Test takers will eliminate answer choices from the guessing pool based on a hunch or intuition. Simple but correct answers often get excluded, leaving a 0% chance of being correct. The monkey has no clue, and often gets lucky with the best choice.

This is why the process of elimination endorsed by most test courses is flawed and detrimental to your performance. Test takers don't guess; they make an ignorant stab in the dark that is usually worse than random.

$5 Challenge

Let me introduce one of the most valuable ideas of this course—the $5 challenge:

You only mark your "best guess" if you are willing to bet $5 on it.
You only eliminate choices from guessing if you are willing to bet $5 on it.

Why $5? Five dollars is an amount of money that is small yet not insignificant, and can really add up fast (20 questions could cost you $100). Likewise, each answer choice on one question of the test will have a small impact on your overall score, but it can really add up to a lot of points in the end.

The process of elimination IS valuable. The following shows your chance of guessing it right:

If you eliminate wrong answer choices until only this many remain:	Chance of getting it correct:
1	100%
2	50%
3	33%

However, if you accidentally eliminate the right answer or go on a hunch for an incorrect answer, your chances drop dramatically—to 0%. By guessing among all the answer choices, you are GUARANTEED to have a shot at the right answer.

That's why the $5 test is so valuable. If you give up the advantage and safety of a pure guess, it had better be worth the risk.

What we still haven't covered is how to be sure that whatever guess you make is truly random. Here's the easiest way:

Always pick the first answer choice among those remaining.

Such a technique means that you have decided, **before you see a single test question**, exactly how you are going to guess, and since the order of choices tells you nothing about which one is correct, this guessing technique is perfectly random.

This section is not meant to scare you away from making educated guesses or eliminating choices; you just need to define when a choice is worth eliminating. The $5 test, along with a pre-defined random guessing strategy, is the best way to make sure you reap all of the benefits of guessing.

Secret Key #3 - Practice Smarter, Not Harder

Many test takers delay the test preparation process because they dread the awful amounts of practice time they think necessary to succeed on the test. We have refined an effective method that will take you only a fraction of the time.

There are a number of "obstacles" in the path to success. Among these are answering questions, finishing in time, and mastering test-taking strategies. All must be executed on the day of the test at peak performance, or your score will suffer. The test is a mental marathon that has a large impact on your future.

Just like a marathon runner, it is important to work your way up to the full challenge. So first you just worry about questions, and then time, and finally strategy:

Success Strategy

1. Find a good source for practice tests.
2. If you are willing to make a larger time investment, consider using more than one study guide. Often the different approaches of multiple authors will help you "get" difficult concepts.
3. Take a practice test with no time constraints, with all study helps, "open book." Take your time with questions and focus on applying strategies.
4. Take a practice test with time constraints, with all guides, "open book."
5. Take a final practice test without open material and with time limits.

If you have time to take more practice tests, just repeat step 5. By gradually exposing yourself to the full rigors of the test environment, you will condition your mind to the stress of test day and maximize your success.

Secret Key #4 - Prepare, Don't Procrastinate

Let me state an obvious fact: if you take the test three times, you will probably get three different scores. This is due to the way you feel on test day, the level of preparedness you have, and the version of the test you see. Despite the test writers' claims to the contrary, some versions of the test WILL be easier for you than others.

Since your future depends so much on your score, you should maximize your chances of success. In order to maximize the likelihood of success, you've got to prepare in advance. This means taking practice tests and spending time learning the information and test taking strategies you will need to succeed.

Never go take the actual test as a "practice" test, expecting that you can just take it again if you need to. Take all the practice tests you can on your own, but when you go to take the official test, be prepared, be focused, and do your best the first time!

Secret Key #5 - Test Yourself

Everyone knows that time is money. There is no need to spend too much of your time or too little of your time preparing for the test. You should only spend as much of your precious time preparing as is necessary for you to get the score you need.

Once you have taken a practice test under real conditions of time constraints, then you will know if you are ready for the test or not.

If you have scored extremely high the first time that you take the practice test, then there is not much point in spending countless hours studying. You are already there.

Benchmark your abilities by retaking practice tests and seeing how much you have improved. Once you consistently score high enough to guarantee success, then you are ready.

If you have scored well below where you need, then knuckle down and begin studying in earnest. Check your improvement regularly through the use of practice tests under real conditions. Above all, don't worry, panic, or give up. The key is perseverance!

Then, when you go to take the test, remain confident and remember how well you did on the practice tests. If you can score high enough on a practice test, then you can do the same on the real thing.

General Strategies

The most important thing you can do is to ignore your fears and jump into the test immediately. Do not be overwhelmed by any strange-sounding terms. You have to jump into the test like jumping into a pool—all at once is the easiest way.

Make Predictions

As you read and understand the question, try to guess what the answer will be. Remember that several of the answer choices are wrong, and once you begin reading them, your mind will immediately become cluttered with answer choices designed to throw you off. Your mind is typically the most focused immediately after you have read the question and digested its contents. If you can, try to predict what the correct answer will be. You may be surprised at what you can predict.

Quickly scan the choices and see if your prediction is in the listed answer choices. If it is, then you can be quite confident that you have the right answer. It still won't hurt to check the other answer choices, but most of the time, you've got it!

Answer the Question

It may seem obvious to only pick answer choices that answer the question, but the test writers can create some excellent answer choices that are wrong. Don't pick an answer just because it sounds right, or you believe it to be true. It MUST answer the question. Once you've made your selection, always go back and check it against the question and make sure that you didn't misread the question and that the answer choice does answer the question posed.

Benchmark

After you read the first answer choice, decide if you think it sounds correct or not. If it doesn't, move on to the next answer choice. If it does, mentally mark that answer choice. This doesn't mean that you've definitely selected it as your answer choice, it just means that it's the best you've seen thus far. Go ahead and read the next choice. If the next choice is worse than the one you've already selected, keep going to the next answer choice. If the next choice is better than the choice you've already selected, mentally mark the new answer choice as your best guess.

The first answer choice that you select becomes your standard. Every other answer choice must be benchmarked against that standard. That choice is correct until proven otherwise by another answer choice beating it out. Once you've decided that no other answer choice seems as good, do one final check to ensure that your answer choice answers the question posed.

Valid Information

Don't discount any of the information provided in the question. Every piece of information may be necessary to determine the correct answer. None of the information in the question is there to throw you off (while the answer choices will certainly have information to throw you off). If two seemingly unrelated topics are discussed, don't ignore either. You can be confident there is a relationship, or it wouldn't be included in the question, and you are probably going to have to determine what is that relationship to find the answer.

Avoid "Fact Traps"

Don't get distracted by a choice that is factually true. Your search is for the answer that answers the question. Stay focused and don't fall for an answer that is true but irrelevant. Always go back to the question and make sure you're choosing an answer that actually answers the question and is not just a true statement. An answer can be factually correct, but it MUST answer the question asked. Additionally, two answers can both be seemingly correct, so be sure to read all of the answer choices, and make sure that you get the one that BEST answers the question.

Milk the Question

Some of the questions may throw you completely off. They might deal with a subject you have not been exposed to, or one that you haven't reviewed in years. While your lack of knowledge about the subject will be a hindrance, the question itself can give you many clues that will help you find the correct answer. Read the question carefully and look for clues. Watch particularly for adjectives and nouns describing difficult terms or words that you don't recognize. Regardless of whether you completely understand a word or not, replacing it with a synonym, either provided or one you more familiar with, may help you to understand what the questions are asking. Rather than wracking your mind about specific detailed information concerning a difficult term or word, try to use mental substitutes that are easier to understand.

The Trap of Familiarity

Don't just choose a word because you recognize it. On difficult questions, you may not recognize a number of words in the answer choices. The test writers don't put "make-believe" words on the test, so don't think that just because you only recognize all the words in one answer choice that that answer choice must be correct. If you only recognize words in one answer choice, then focus on that one. Is it correct? Try your best to determine if it is correct. If it is, that's great. If not, eliminate it. Each word and answer choice you eliminate increases your chances of getting the question correct, even if you then have to guess among the unfamiliar choices.

Eliminate Answers

Eliminate choices as soon as you realize they are wrong. But be careful! Make sure you consider all of the possible answer choices. Just because one appears right, doesn't mean that the next one won't be even better! The test writers will usually put more than one good answer choice for every question, so read all of them. Don't worry if you are stuck between two that seem right. By getting down to just two remaining possible choices, your odds are now 50/50. Rather than wasting too much time, play the odds. You are guessing, but guessing wisely because you've been able to knock out some of the answer choices that you know are wrong. If you are eliminating choices and realize that the last answer choice you are left with is also obviously wrong, don't panic. Start over and consider each choice again. There may easily be something that you missed the first time and will realize on the second pass.

Tough Questions

If you are stumped on a problem or it appears too hard or too difficult, don't waste time. Move on! Remember though, if you can quickly check for obviously incorrect answer choices, your chances of guessing correctly are greatly improved. Before you completely give up, at least try to knock out a couple of possible answers. Eliminate what you can and then guess at the remaining answer choices before moving on.

Brainstorm

If you get stuck on a difficult question, spend a few seconds quickly brainstorming. Run through the complete list of possible answer choices. Look at each choice and ask yourself, "Could this answer the question satisfactorily?" Go through each answer choice and consider it independently of the others. By systematically going through all possibilities, you may find something that you would otherwise overlook. Remember though that when you get stuck, it's important to try to keep moving.

Read Carefully

Understand the problem. Read the question and answer choices carefully. Don't miss the question because you misread the terms. You have plenty of time to read each question thoroughly and make sure you understand what is being asked. Yet a happy medium must be attained, so don't waste too much time. You must read carefully, but efficiently.

Face Value

When in doubt, use common sense. Always accept the situation in the problem at face value. Don't read too much into it. These problems will not require you to make huge leaps of logic. The test writers aren't trying to throw you off with a cheap trick. If you have to go beyond creativity and make a leap of logic in order to have an answer choice answer the question, then you should look at the other answer choices. Don't overcomplicate the problem by creating theoretical relationships or explanations that will warp time or space. These are normal problems rooted in reality. It's just that the applicable relationship or explanation may not be readily apparent and you have to figure things out. Use your common sense to interpret anything that isn't clear.

Prefixes

If you're having trouble with a word in the question or answer choices, try dissecting it. Take advantage of every clue that the word might include. Prefixes and suffixes can be a huge help. Usually they allow you to determine a basic meaning. Pre- means before, post-means after, pro - is positive, de- is negative. From these prefixes and suffixes, you can get an idea of the general meaning of the word and try to put it into context. Beware though of any traps. Just because con- is the opposite of pro-, doesn't necessarily mean congress is the opposite of progress!

Hedge Phrases

Watch out for critical hedge phrases, led off with words such as "likely," "may," "can," "sometimes," "often," "almost," "mostly," "usually," "generally," "rarely," and "sometimes." Question writers insert these hedge phrases to cover every possibility. Often an answer choice will be wrong simply because it leaves no room for exception. Unless the situation calls for them, avoid answer choices that have definitive words like "exactly," and "always."

Switchback Words

Stay alert for "switchbacks." These are the words and phrases frequently used to alert you to shifts in thought. The most common switchback word is "but." Others include "although," "however," "nevertheless," "on the other hand," "even though," "while," "in spite of," "despite," and "regardless of."

New Information

Correct answer choices will rarely have completely new information included. Answer choices typically are straightforward reflections of the material asked about and will directly relate to the question. If a new piece of information is included in an answer choice that doesn't even seem to relate to the topic being asked about, then that answer choice is likely incorrect. All of the information needed to answer the question is usually provided for you in the question. You should not have to make guesses that are unsupported or choose answer choices that require unknown information that cannot be reasoned from what is given.

Time Management

On technical questions, don't get lost on the technical terms. Don't spend too much time on any one question. If you don't know what a term means, then odds are you aren't going to get much further since you don't have a dictionary. You should be able to immediately recognize whether or not you know a term. If you don't, work with the other clues that you have—the other answer choices and terms provided—but don't waste too much time trying to figure out a difficult term that you don't know.

Contextual Clues

Look for contextual clues. An answer can be right but not the correct answer. The contextual clues will help you find the answer that is most right and is correct. Understand the context in which a phrase or statement is made. This will help you make important distinctions.

Don't Panic

Panicking will not answer any questions for you; therefore, it isn't helpful. When you first see the question, if your mind goes blank, take a deep breath. Force yourself to mechanically go through the steps of solving the problem using the strategies you've learned.

Pace Yourself

Don't get clock fever. It's easy to be overwhelmed when you're looking at a page full of questions, your mind is full of random thoughts and feeling confused, and the clock is ticking down faster than you would like. Calm down and maintain the pace that you have set for yourself. As long as you are on track by monitoring your pace, you are guaranteed to have enough time for yourself. When you get to the last few minutes of the test, it may seem like you won't have enough time left, but if you only have as many questions as you should have left at that point, then you're right on track!

Answer Selection

The best way to pick an answer choice is to eliminate all of those that are wrong, until only one is left and confirm that is the correct answer. Sometimes though, an answer choice may immediately look right. Be careful! Take a second to make sure that the other choices are not equally obvious. Don't make a hasty mistake. There are only two times that you should stop before checking other answers. First is when you are positive that the answer choice you have selected is correct. Second is when time is almost out and you have to make a quick guess!

Check Your Work

Since you will probably not know every term listed and the answer to every question, it is important that you get credit for the ones that you do know. Don't miss any questions through careless mistakes. If at all possible, try to take a second to look back over your answer selection and make sure you've selected the correct answer choice and haven't made a costly careless mistake (such as marking an answer choice that you didn't mean to mark). The time it takes for this quick double check should more than pay for itself in caught mistakes.

Beware of Directly Quoted Answers

Sometimes an answer choice will repeat word for word a portion of the question or reference section. However, beware of such exact duplication. It may be a trap! More than likely, the correct choice will paraphrase or summarize a point, rather than being exactly the same wording.

Slang

Scientific sounding answers are better than slang ones. An answer choice that begins "To compare the outcomes…" is much more likely to be correct than one that begins "Because some people insisted…"

Extreme Statements

Avoid wild answers that throw out highly controversial ideas that are proclaimed as established fact. An answer choice that states the "process should be used in certain situations, if…" is much more likely to be correct than one that states the "process should be discontinued completely." The first is a calm rational statement and doesn't even make a definitive, uncompromising stance, using a hedge word "if" to provide wiggle room, whereas the second choice is a radical idea and far more extreme.

Answer Choice Families

When you have two or more answer choices that are direct opposites or parallels, one of them is usually the correct answer. For instance, if one answer choice states "x increases" and another answer choice states "x decreases" or "y increases," then those two or three answer choices are very similar in construction and fall into the same family of answer choices. A family of answer choices consists of two or three answer choices, very similar in construction, but often with directly opposite meanings. Usually the correct answer choice will be in that family of answer choices. The "odd man out" or answer choice that doesn't seem to fit the parallel construction of the other answer choices is more likely to be incorrect.

Special Report: What is Test Anxiety and How to Overcome It?

The very nature of tests caters to some level of anxiety, nervousness, or tension, just as we feel for any important event that occurs in our lives. A little bit of anxiety or nervousness can be a good thing. It helps us with motivation, and makes achievement just that much sweeter. However, too much anxiety can be a problem, especially if it hinders our ability to function and perform.

"Test anxiety," is the term that refers to the emotional reactions that some test-takers experience when faced with a test or exam. Having a fear of testing and exams is based upon a rational fear, since the test-taker's performance can shape the course of an academic career. Nevertheless, experiencing excessive fear of examinations will only interfere with the test-taker's ability to perform and chance to be successful.

There are a large variety of causes that can contribute to the development and sensation of test anxiety. These include, but are not limited to, lack of preparation and worrying about issues surrounding the test.

Lack of Preparation

Lack of preparation can be identified by the following behaviors or situations:

Not scheduling enough time to study, and therefore cramming the night before the test or exam
Managing time poorly, to create the sensation that there is not enough time to do everything
Failing to organize the text information in advance, so that the study material consists of the entire text and not simply the pertinent information
Poor overall studying habits

Worrying, on the other hand, can be related to both the test taker, or many other factors around him/her that will be affected by the results of the test. These include worrying about:

Previous performances on similar exams, or exams in general
How friends and other students are achieving
The negative consequences that will result from a poor grade or failure

There are three primary elements to test anxiety. Physical components, which involve the same typical bodily reactions as those to acute anxiety (to be discussed below). Emotional factors have to do with fear or panic. Mental or cognitive issues concerning attention spans and memory abilities.

Physical Signals

There are many different symptoms of test anxiety, and these are not limited to mental and emotional strain. Frequently there are a range of physical signals that will let a test taker know that he/she is suffering from test anxiety. These bodily changes can include the following:

Perspiring
Sweaty palms
Wet, trembling hands
Nausea
Dry mouth
A knot in the stomach
Headache
Faintness
Muscle tension
Aching shoulders, back and neck
Rapid heart beat
Feeling too hot/cold

To recognize the sensation of test anxiety, a test-taker should monitor him/herself for the following sensations:

The physical distress symptoms as listed above
Emotional sensitivity, expressing emotional feelings such as the need to cry or laugh too much, or a sensation of anger or helplessness
A decreased ability to think, causing the test-taker to blank out or have racing thoughts that are hard to organize or control.

Though most students will feel some level of anxiety when faced with a test or exam, the majority can cope with that anxiety and maintain it at a manageable level. However, those who cannot are faced with a very real and very serious condition, which can and should be controlled for the immeasurable benefit of this sufferer.

Naturally, these sensations lead to negative results for the testing experience. The most common effects of test anxiety have to do with nervousness and mental blocking.

Nervousness

Nervousness can appear in several different levels:

The test-taker's difficulty, or even inability to read and understand the questions on the test
The difficulty or inability to organize thoughts to a coherent form
The difficulty or inability to recall key words and concepts relating to the testing questions (especially essays)
The receipt of poor grades on a test, though the test material was well known by the test taker

Conversely, a person may also experience mental blocking, which involves:

Blanking out on test questions
Only remembering the correct answers to the questions when the test has already finished.

Fortunately for test anxiety sufferers, beating these feelings, to a large degree, has to do with proper preparation. When a test taker has a feeling of preparedness, then anxiety will be dramatically lessened.

The first step to resolving anxiety issues is to distinguish which of the two types of anxiety are being suffered. If the anxiety is a direct result of a lack of preparation, this should be considered a normal reaction, and the anxiety level (as opposed to the test results) shouldn't be anything to worry about. However, if, when adequately prepared, the test-taker still panics, blanks out, or seems to overreact, this is not a fully rational reaction. While this can be considered normal too, there are many ways to combat and overcome these effects.

Remember that anxiety cannot be entirely eliminated, however, there are ways to minimize it, to make the anxiety easier to manage. Preparation is one of the best ways to minimize test anxiety. Therefore the following techniques are wise in order to best fight off any anxiety that may want to build.

To begin with, try to avoid cramming before a test, whenever it is possible. By trying to memorize an entire term's worth of information in one day, you'll be shocking your system, and not giving yourself a very good chance to absorb the information. This is an easy path to anxiety, so for those who suffer from test anxiety, cramming should not even be considered an option.

Instead of cramming, work throughout the semester to combine all of the material which is presented throughout the semester, and work on it gradually as the course goes by, making sure to master the main concepts first, leaving minor details for a week or so before the test.

To study for the upcoming exam, be sure to pose questions that may be on the examination, to gauge the ability to answer them by integrating the ideas from your texts, notes and lectures, as well as any supplementary readings.

If it is truly impossible to cover all of the information that was covered in that particular term, concentrate on the most important portions, that can be covered very well. Learn these concepts as best as possible, so that when the test comes, a goal can be made to use these concepts as presentations of your knowledge.

In addition to study habits, changes in attitude are critical to beating a struggle with test anxiety. In fact, an improvement of the perspective over the entire test-taking experience can actually help a test taker to enjoy studying and therefore improve the overall experience. Be certain not to overemphasize the significance of the grade - know that the result of the test is neither a reflection of self worth, nor is it a measure of intelligence; one grade will not predict a person's future success.

To improve an overall testing outlook, the following steps should be tried:

Keeping in mind that the most reasonable expectation for taking a test is to expect to try to demonstrate as much of what you know as you possibly can.

Reminding ourselves that a test is only one test, this is not the only one, and there will be others.

The thought of thinking of oneself in an irrational, all-or-nothing term should be avoided at all costs.

A reward should be designated for after the test, so there's something to look forward to. Whether it be going to a movie, going out to eat, or simply visiting friends, schedule it in advance, and do it no matter what result is expected on the exam.

Test-takers should also keep in mind that the basics are some of the most important things, even beyond anti-anxiety techniques and studying. Never neglect the basic social, emotional and biological needs, in order to try to absorb information. In order to best achieve, these three factors must be held as just as important as the studying itself.

Study Steps

Remember the following important steps for studying:

Maintain healthy nutrition and exercise habits. Continue both your recreational activities and social pass times. These both contribute to your physical and emotional well being.

Be certain to get a good amount of sleep, especially the night before the test, because when you're overtired you are not able to perform to the best of your best ability.

Keep the studying pace to a moderate level by taking breaks when they are needed, and varying the work whenever possible, to keep the mind fresh instead of getting bored.

When enough studying has been done that all the material that can be learned has been learned, and the test taker is prepared for the test, stop studying and do something relaxing such as listening to music, watching a movie, or taking a warm bubble bath.

There are also many other techniques to minimize the uneasiness or apprehension that is experienced along with test anxiety before, during, or even after the examination. In fact, there are a great deal of things that can be done to stop anxiety from interfering with lifestyle and performance. Again, remember that anxiety will not be eliminated entirely, and it shouldn't be. Otherwise that "up" feeling for exams would not exist, and most of us depend on that sensation to perform better than usual. However, this anxiety has to be at a level that is manageable.

Of course, as we have just discussed, being prepared for the exam is half the battle right away. Attending all classes, finding out what knowledge will be expected on the exam, and knowing the exam schedules are easy steps to lowering anxiety. Keeping up with work will remove the need to cram, and efficient study habits will eliminate wasted time. Studying should be done in an ideal location for concentration, so that it is simple to become interested in the material and give it complete attention. A method such as SQ3R (Survey, Question, Read, Recite, Review) is a wonderful key to follow to make sure that the study habits are as effective as possible, especially in the case of learning from a textbook. Flashcards are great techniques for memorization. Learning to take good notes will mean that notes will be full of useful information, so that less sifting will need to be done to seek out what is pertinent for studying. Reviewing notes after class and then again on occasion will keep the information fresh in the mind. From notes that have been taken summary sheets and outlines can be made for simpler reviewing.

A study group can also be a very motivational and helpful place to study, as there will be a sharing of ideas, all of the minds can work together, to make sure that everyone understands, and the studying will be made more interesting because it will be a social occasion.

Basically, though, as long as the test-taker remains organized and self confident, with efficient study habits, less time will need to be spent studying, and higher grades will be achieved.

To become self confident, there are many useful steps. The first of these is "self talk." It has been shown through extensive research, that self-talk for students who suffer from test anxiety, should be well monitored, in order to make sure that it contributes to self confidence as opposed to sinking the student. Frequently the self talk of test-anxious students is negative or self-defeating, thinking that everyone else is smarter and faster, that they always mess up, and that if they don't do well, they'll fail the entire course. It is important to decreasing anxiety that awareness is made of self talk. Try writing any negative self thoughts and then disputing them with a positive statement instead. Begin self-encouragement as though it was a friend speaking. Repeat positive statements to help reprogram the mind to believing in successes instead of failures.

Helpful Techniques

Other extremely helpful techniques include:

Self-visualization of doing well and reaching goals
While aiming for an "A" level of understanding, don't try to "overprotect" by setting your expectations lower. This will only convince the mind to stop studying in order to meet the lower expectations.
Don't make comparisons with the results or habits of other students. These are individual factors, and different things work for different people, causing different results.
Strive to become an expert in learning what works well, and what can be done in order to improve. Consider collecting this data in a journal.
Create rewards for after studying instead of doing things before studying that will only turn into avoidance behaviors.
Make a practice of relaxing - by using methods such as progressive relaxation, self-hypnosis, guided imagery, etc - in order to make relaxation an automatic sensation.
Work on creating a state of relaxed concentration so that concentrating will take on the focus of the mind, so that none will be wasted on worrying.
Take good care of the physical self by eating well and getting enough sleep.
Plan in time for exercise and stick to this plan.

Beyond these techniques, there are other methods to be used before, during and after the test that will help the test-taker perform well in addition to overcoming anxiety.

Before the exam comes the academic preparation. This involves establishing a study schedule and beginning at least one week before the actual date of the test. By doing this, the anxiety of not having enough time to study for the test will be automatically eliminated. Moreover, this will make the studying a much more effective experience, ensuring that the learning will be an easier process. This relieves much undue pressure on the test-taker.

Summary sheets, note cards, and flash cards with the main concepts and examples of these main concepts should be prepared in advance of the actual studying time. A topic should never be eliminated from this process. By omitting a topic because it isn't expected to be on the test is only setting up the test-taker for anxiety should it actually appear on the exam. Utilize the course syllabus for laying out the topics that should be studied. Carefully go over the notes that were made in class, paying special attention to any of the issues that the professor took special care to emphasize while lecturing in class. In the textbooks, use the chapter review, or if possible, the chapter tests, to begin your review.

It may even be possible to ask the instructor what information will be covered on the exam, or what the format of the exam will be (for example, multiple choice, essay, free form, true-false). Additionally, see if it is possible to find out how many questions will be on the test. If a review sheet or sample test has been offered by the professor, make good use of it, above anything else, for the preparation for the test. Another great resource for getting to know the examination is reviewing tests from previous semesters. Use these tests to review, and aim to achieve a 100% score on each of the possible topics. With a few exceptions, the goal that you set for yourself is the highest one that you will reach.

Take all of the questions that were assigned as homework, and rework them to any other possible course material. The more problems reworked, the more skill and confidence will form as a result. When forming the solution to a problem, write out each of the steps. Don't simply do head work. By doing as many steps on paper as possible, much clarification and therefore confidence will be formed. Do this with as many homework problems as possible, before checking the answers. By checking the answer after each problem, a reinforcement will exist, that will not be on the exam. Study situations should be as exam-like as possible, to prime the test-taker's system for the experience. By waiting to check the answers at the end, a psychological advantage will be formed, to decrease the stress factor.

Another fantastic reason for not cramming is the avoidance of confusion in concepts, especially when it comes to mathematics. 8-10 hours of study will become one hundred percent more effective if it is spread out over a week or at least several days, instead of doing it all in one sitting. Recognize that the human brain requires time in order to assimilate new material, so frequent breaks and a span of study time over several days will be much more beneficial.

Additionally, don't study right up until the point of the exam. Studying should stop a minimum of one hour before the exam begins. This allows the brain to rest and put things in their proper order. This will also provide the time to become as relaxed as possible when going into the examination room. The test-taker will also have time to eat well and eat sensibly. Know that the brain needs food as much as the rest of the body. With enough food and enough sleep, as well as a relaxed attitude, the body and the mind are primed for success.

Avoid any anxious classmates who are talking about the exam. These students only spread anxiety, and are not worth sharing the anxious sentimentalities.

Before the test also involves creating a positive attitude, so mental preparation should also be a point of concentration. There are many keys to creating a positive attitude. Should fears become rushing in, make a visualization of taking the exam, doing well, and seeing an A written on the paper. Write out a list of affirmations that will bring a feeling of confidence, such as "I am doing well in my English class," "I studied well and know my material," "I enjoy this class."

Even if the affirmations aren't believed at first, it sends a positive message to the subconscious which will result in an alteration of the overall belief system, which is the system that creates reality.

If a sensation of panic begins, work with the fear and imagine the very worst! Work through the entire scenario of not passing the test, failing the entire course, and dropping out of school, followed by not getting a job, and pushing a shopping cart through the dark alley where you'll live. This will place things into perspective! Then, practice deep breathing and create a visualization of the opposite situation - achieving an "A" on the exam, passing the entire course, receiving the degree at a graduation ceremony.

On the day of the test, there are many things to be done to ensure the best results, as well as the most calm outlook. The following stages are suggested in order to maximize test-taking potential:

Begin the examination day with a moderate breakfast, and avoid any coffee or beverages with caffeine if the test taker is prone to jitters. Even people who are used to managing caffeine can feel jittery or light-headed when it is taken on a test day.
Attempt to do something that is relaxing before the examination begins. As last minute cramming clouds the mastering of overall concepts, it is better to use this time to create a calming outlook.
Be certain to arrive at the test location well in advance, in order to provide time to select a location that is away from doors, windows and other distractions, as well as giving enough time to relax before the test begins.
Keep away from anxiety generating classmates who will upset the sensation of stability and relaxation that is being attempted before the exam.
Should the waiting period before the exam begins cause anxiety, create a self-distraction by reading a light magazine or something else that is relaxing and simple.

During the exam itself, read the entire exam from beginning to end, and find out how much time should be allotted to each individual problem. Once writing the exam, should more time be taken for a problem, it should be abandoned, in order to begin another problem. If there is time at the end, the unfinished problem can always be returned to and completed.

Read the instructions very carefully - twice - so that unpleasant surprises won't follow during or after the exam has ended.

When writing the exam, pretend that the situation is actually simply the completion of homework within a library, or at home. This will assist in forming a relaxed atmosphere, and will allow the brain extra focus for the complex thinking function.

Begin the exam with all of the questions with which the most confidence is felt. This will build the confidence level regarding the entire exam and will begin a quality momentum. This will also create encouragement for trying the problems where uncertainty resides.

Going with the "gut instinct" is always the way to go when solving a problem. Second guessing should be avoided at all costs. Have confidence in the ability to do well.

For **essay questions**, create an outline in advance that will keep the mind organized and make certain that all of the points are remembered. For multiple choice, read every answer, even if the correct one has been spotted - a better one may exist.

Continue at a pace that is reasonable and not rushed, in order to be able to work carefully. Provide enough time to go over the answers at the end, to check for small errors that can be corrected.

Should a feeling of panic begin, breathe deeply, and think of the feeling of the body releasing sand through its pores. Visualize a calm, peaceful place, and include all of the sights, sounds and sensations of this image. Continue the deep breathing, and take a few minutes to continue this with closed eyes. When all is well again, return to the test.

If a "blanking" occurs for a certain question, skip it and move on to the next question. There will be time to return to the other question later. Get everything done that can be done, first, to guarantee all the grades that can be compiled, and to build all of the confidence possible. Then return to the weaker questions to build the marks from there.

Remember, one's own reality can be created, so as long as the belief is there, success will follow. And remember: anxiety can happen later, right now, there's an exam to be written!

After the examination is complete, whether there is a feeling for a good grade or a bad grade, don't dwell on the exam, and be certain to follow through on the reward that was promised...and enjoy it! Don't dwell on any mistakes that have been made, as there is nothing that can be done at this point anyway.

Additionally, don't begin to study for the next test right away. Do something relaxing for a while, and let the mind relax and prepare itself to begin absorbing information again.

From the results of the exam - both the grade and the entire experience, be certain to learn from what has gone on. Perfect studying habits and work some more on confidence in order to make the next examination experience even better than the last one.

Learn to avoid places where openings occurred for laziness, procrastination and day dreaming.

Use the time between this exam and the next one to better learn to relax, even learning to relax on cue, so that any anxiety can be controlled during the next exam. Learn how to relax the body. Slouch in your chair if that helps. Tighten and then relax all of the different muscle groups, one group at a time, beginning with the feet and then working all the way up to the neck and face. This will ultimately relax the muscles more than they were to begin with. Learn how to breathe deeply and comfortably, and focus on this breathing going in and out as a relaxing thought. With every exhale, repeat the word "relax."

As common as test anxiety is, it is very possible to overcome it. Make yourself one of the test-takers who overcome this frustrating hindrance.

Special Report: Retaking the Test: What Are Your Chances at Improving Your Score?

After going through the experience of taking a major test, many test takers feel that once is enough. The test usually comes during a period of transition in the test taker's life, and taking the test is only one of a series of important events. With so many distractions and conflicting recommendations, it may be difficult for a test taker to rationally determine whether or not he should retake the test after viewing his scores.

The importance of the test usually only adds to the burden of the retake decision. However, don't be swayed by emotion. There a few simple questions that you can ask yourself to guide you as you try to determine whether a retake would improve your score:

1. What went wrong? Why wasn't your score what you expected?

Can you point to a single factor or problem that you feel caused the low score? Were you sick on test day? Was there an emotional upheaval in your life that caused a distraction? Were you late for the test or not able to use the full time allotment? If you can point to any of these specific, individual problems, then a retake should definitely be considered.

2. Is there enough time to improve?

Many problems that may show up in your score report may take a lot of time for improvement. A deficiency in a particular math skill may require weeks or months of tutoring and studying to improve. If you have enough time to improve an identified weakness, then a retake should definitely be considered.

3. How will additional scores be used? Will a score average, highest score, or most recent score be used?

Different test scores may be handled completely differently. If you've taken the test multiple times, sometimes your highest score is used, sometimes your average score is computed and used, and sometimes your most recent score is used. Make sure you understand what method will be used to evaluate your scores, and use that to help you determine whether a retake should be considered.

4. Are my practice test scores significantly higher than my actual test score?

If you have taken a lot of practice tests and are consistently scoring at a much higher level than your actual test score, then you should consider a retake. However, if you've taken five practice tests and only one of your scores was higher than your actual test score, or if your practice test scores were only slightly higher than your actual test score, then it is unlikely that you will significantly increase your score.

5. Do I need perfect scores or will I be able to live with this score? Will this score still allow me to follow my dreams?

What kind of score is acceptable to you? Is your current score "good enough?" Do you have to have a certain score in order to pursue the future of your dreams? If you won't be happy with your current score, and there's no way that you could live with it, then you should consider a retake. However, don't get your hopes up. If you are looking for significant improvement, that may or may not be possible. But if you won't be happy otherwise, it is at least worth the effort. Remember that there are other considerations. To achieve your dream, it is likely that your grades may also be taken into account. A great test score is usually not the only thing necessary to succeed. Make sure that you aren't overemphasizing the importance of a high test score.

Furthermore, a retake does not always result in a higher score. Some test takers will score lower on a retake, rather than higher. One study shows that one-fourth of test takers will achieve a significant improvement in test score, while one-sixth of test takers will actually show a decrease. While this shows that most test takers will improve, the majority will only improve their scores a little and a retake may not be worth the test taker's effort.

Finally, if a test is taken only once and is considered in the added context of good grades on the part of a test taker, the person reviewing the grades and scores may be tempted to assume that the test taker just had a bad day while taking the test, and may discount the low test score in favor of the high grades. But if the test is retaken and the scores are approximately the same, then the validity of the low scores are only confirmed. Therefore, a retake could actually hurt a test taker by definitely bracketing a test taker's score ability to a limited range.

Special Report: Additional Bonus Material

Due to our efforts to try to keep this book to a manageable length, we've created a link that will give you access to all of your additional bonus material.

Please visit http://www.mometrix.com/bonus948/chpna to access the information.